Your **Guide** to

OIL OF OREGANO

Better Health for **People** & **Pets**

Tracy K. Gibbs, PhD

MANNAFEST PUBLISHING INC.

4 - 740 Waddington Drive
Vernon, B.C. V1T 9E9
Canada

Printed in China

Published by:
Mannafest Publishing Inc.
4 - 740 Waddington Drive
Vernon, B.C. V1T 9E9 Canada

Design and Layout:
John Skipp / Creative Licence Design

Copyright © 2013 by Mannafest Publishing Inc.

ISBN 978-0-9919788-0-9

Paper sourced from sustainably managed forests.

Disclaimer: The information in this booklet is provided with the understanding that the author is not engaged in rendering medical advice. It is provided for educational purposes only and is not intended as a diagnosis, treatment, cure, or prevention of any health condition. Consult a healthcare professional for advice. The decision to use, or not to use, any of this information is the sole responsibility of the reader.

Contents

Part 5 - Success with Oil of Oregano 91

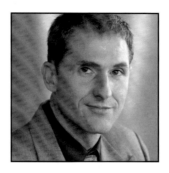

About the Author

Tracy K. Gibbs, Ph.D., has an extensive background in pharmacognosy, the study of medicines derived from natural sources. He studied chemistry, hematology and botanical medicine in Japan. Upon returning to the U.S., he enrolled in nutritional classes at Clayton College of Natural Health and studied iridology under Dr. Bernard Jensen. He also studied at the College of Naturopathic Medicine and Surgery, where he currently teaches classes in Pharmacognosy and Botanical Medicine. He is a member of the International Iridology Practitioners Association (IIPA), a board member in the International Health Food Research Foundation in Nagoya, Japan, and a member of the American Society of Pharmacognosy.

Dr. Gibbs has lectured all over the world on the clinical applications of herbal medicine and has unique insights on the future innovation of herb-based drugs in the U.S. He operates schools in both Japan and the U.S., teaching people how to use herbs in everyday situations as an alternative to visiting crowded medical clinics.

Dr. Gibbs has authored several books and booklets, including *My Home Pharmacy, Enzyme Power, Phytonutrients: The Drugs of the Future,* and *Your Blood Speaks.* Two of these books have been printed in Japanese. He also completed the first English textbook on performing Live Cell Morphology, using methods that have been approved in other countries.

Currently, Dr. Gibbs is the owner and founder of Health Education Corporation, specializing in nutritional blood evaluation, educational seminars, literature production and personal counseling. He is also a co-owner and chief formulator for NutraNomics, Inc., a Salt Lake City-based corporation involved in the research and development of nutritional supplements and herbal products.

Foreword

As a young child, on a visit to my aunt's home in Modesto, California, I had an experience that was to have a lasting impact on my life and career. While my mother and her sister were talking, I wandered into the backyard and noticed a beautiful cherry tree. Coming from the colder climate of Idaho, where our cherry trees never grew very tall, I was fascinated not only by the size of the tree, but also by the wonderfully dark, red cherries hanging high overhead. After climbing halfway to the top and finding a comfortable spot, I began to pluck the cherries one by one, and for the rest of that morning I enjoyed a veritable feast of that sweet, ripe fruit. It wasn't long after getting down from that tree that I discovered an interesting side effect of eating too many cherries. Let's just say that I became very well acquainted with my aunt's bathroom that afternoon...

That experience was one of many that led me to question why certain foods affect our bodies the way they do. Each and every food item has an effect. Most are positive and help our bodies grow and become strong. Many fight diseases and help build our immune systems. A few, however, have negative consequences. Morgan Spurlock explored this common-sense principle in his documentary *Super Size Me*, in which he decided to experiment with his own body by eating exclusively at McDonalds for 30 days. Within three weeks, the 32-year-old gained almost 25 pounds, increased his body mass by 13 percent, and nearly destroyed his liver!

The current policy of the U.S. Food and Drug Administration (FDA) is that foods are "neutral"; i.e., they cannot make you sick, and they certainly cannot make you healthy. The Federal Trade Commission (FTC) does not allow food labels to say, "This food is good for you" or "This food is bad for you," and no claims can be made on any food that may indicate a particular health benefit or side effect. Can you imagine if the FTC mandated a label for cherries stating, "Warning: Overconsumption may cause diarrhea" that had to be stickered on each individual cherry? How about a warning on grapefruits which read, "Warning: May cause your liver to block certain medications"? Personally, I would love to see a sticker on an apple that read, "An apple a day keeps the doctor away!" or on a pomegranate that read, "Attention: Contains active compounds that may help prevent cancer and heart disease." If the FTC and FDA allowed these types of claims, our produce sections and farmers' markets would be more like pharmacies, with registered botanists behind every counter warning us of the side effects or possible health benefits of each food item.

So why do certain foods have the ability to change our health and alter normal metabolic processes in our bodies? We know that all foods contain vitamins, minerals, proteins, fats, fiber, and sugars, but these are just simple building blocks that our bodies use as raw materials to maintain normal functioning of all our systems and organs. What gives a certain food the ability to fight a cold or another the ability to give us energy? What is it in chocolate that gives us that happy feeling? What is in cayenne pepper that causes our body temperature to rise?

There is indisputable evidence proving that whole, unadulterated plants (and their roots, stems, leaves, flowers, fruits, nuts and seeds) contain active chemicals. These active ingredients are known as phytochemicals (plant-based natural chemicals). Phytochemicals are not man-made but are found naturally in every plant on this planet. Some phytochemicals are deadly toxins, some have been proven to cure cancer, and some hold the keys to longevity. Thousands of others still hide their mysteries, waiting for some enterprising scientist to unlock their secrets. Without specific knowledge of their cellular actions or mechanisms, herbal plants and their phytochemicals have been used as medicine for millennia. For example, Hippocrates prescribed willow tree leaves to abate fever. Much later, the phytochemical Salicin was extracted from willow tree bark and synthetically produced as the familiar drug, aspirin. Many of our pharmaceutical drugs today are re-created, synthetic derivatives of phytochemicals that were originally found in plants.

Commonly known herbs, vegetables, leafy greens, fruits, nuts and seeds are all ripe with beneficial, active phytochemicals that are known to improve health, boost immunity, fight disease and prevent the onset of illness. Since each of these foods is unique in its chemistry, each will work differently and have its own strengths, or effects. Of all the different foods you can find in your local produce section, there is one that stands out for its medicinal uses. That remarkable food is the subject of this book: Oregano.

As you will discover, oregano's greatest gift is its ability to fight off infections, which are a leading cause of illness and disease worldwide. At a time in history when conventional treatments are no longer working and drug companies have thrown in the towel, the need for oregano and its essential oil has never been greater.

1

Antibiotics, Our Children, Our Planet

Infectious Disease

Infections are a leading cause of death, disability and illness worldwide. They result when pathogenic microorganisms—bacteria, viruses, parasites, fungi, or protozoa—invade and colonize in the body and manifest as disease. The body has its own natural defenses, and many infections are often short-lived. But in the past 30 years, the growing virulence of pathogens has caused a rise in hospitalizations and deaths.

Some infections are acute and cause severe illness, while other infections can remain in the body for years, manifesting as chronic, degenerative diseases that are typically referred to as "non-communicable diseases" (NCDs). In 2008, the World Health Organization (WHO) estimates that 36 million people died of NCDs, roughly two-thirds of annual fatalities worldwide.[1] In recent years, the growing incidence of NCDs is being referred to as a global pandemic.

The sobering fact is that infections are responsible, directly or indirectly, for tens of millions of deaths every year, as well as millions of disabilities. HIV, malaria, diarrhea, measles, pneumonia and tuberculosis are at the top of the list, but numerous other infectious diseases pose a growing concern today. To make matters worse, young children and the elderly are most at risk.

Antimicrobial Resistance: A Growing Concern

There was a time in history when antibiotics were hailed as miracle drugs. With the introduction of penicillin in the 1940s, and the subsequent discovery of streptomycin, the world saw a dramatic reduction in illness and death from infectious diseases. However, the battle of the bugs was far from over. Disease-causing organisms (a.k.a. infectious microbes or pathogens) have the ability to mutate and acquire resistant genes from other organisms and thereby develop resistance to drugs. Take the example of *Staphylococcus aureus*, a common cause of hospital infections. As early as 1942, staph infection began to show resistance to penicillin, and 20 years later, more than 80 percent of staph bacteria were penicillin-resistant. Though antimicrobial resistance (AMR) is not a new phenomenon, it has increased dramatically in the past 20 years and now poses a serious threat to the treatment of infections. Pathogens that are rapidly developing resistance to available treatments include the bacteria that cause pneumonia, ear infections, meningitis and sinusitis (i.e. *Streptococcus pneumonia*); skin, heart, bone, lung and bloodstream infections (i.e. *Staphylococcus aureus*); urinary tract infections (i.e. *Escherichia coli)*; sexually transmitted diseases (i.e. *Neisseria gonorrhoeae*); foodborne infections (i.e. *Salmonella* and *E. coli*); intestinal infections (*Clostridium difficile*); and infections transmitted in healthcare settings (i.e. *Enterococcus ssp.*, *Acinetobacter baumanii*, *Pseudomonas aeruginosa*, and *Klebsiella spp.*).

While bacteria are the most common cause of infectious disease-related deaths, resistance is prevalent in all classes of pathogens: viruses, fungi, parasites and protozoa. For instance, the viruses that cause influenza, hepatitis B and HIV; the fungi that cause yeast infections; the parasites that cause malaria; and the protozoa that cause giardiasis, are all developing increased resistance to current treatments. This makes perfect sense, since all organisms are subject to natural selection. Antimicrobial resistance is simply the natural process of adaptation and micro-evolution, where drugs increase selective pressure, encouraging resistant strains to thrive and more susceptible strains to die off.

Some pathogens have resistance to a single antimicrobial drug (or class of drugs), while others are resistant to several drugs (or classes). The latter are referred to as multidrug-resistant (MDR) strains, or more commonly "superbugs." In some cases, these pesky pathogens have become so resistant that even the newest, third-generation, broad-spectrum antibiotics have proven ineffective. For example, *Acinetobacter baumannii*, *Pseudomonas aeruginosa*, *Klebsiella pneumonia* and *Escherichia coli* have all shown an increasing resistance to newer cephalosporins, fluoroquinolones, and aminoglycosides.[2] In response, the medical community has resorted to a restricted class of "last-line" antibiotics called carbapenems, but even that line is under siege. The incidence of carbapenem-resistant bacterial infections is already disturbingly high in some countries, with outbreaks being reported. What is more concerning is there are currently no new antibiotics in the pipeline to treat the superbugs resistant to carbapenems; authorities state that the worldwide spread of the resistance gene is a potential nightmare scenario.[3]

Vancomycin is another example of a powerful, last-line antibiotic that is losing its effectiveness against the very bacteria it has helped to create. Used successfully in hospital settings since 1958, Vancomycin became a standard treatment in the 1980s for pseudomembranous colitis, and drug-resistant bacteria like methicillin-resistant Staphylococcus aureus (MRSA). But due to its overuse, bacteria such as Enterococcus and MRSA developed resistance to Vancomycin (VRE and VRSA) and today are responsible for thousands of deaths annually.[4]

Hospital-Acquired Infections (HAI)

Patients in hospitals and health-care facilities are at the highest risk of contracting multidrug-resistant infections. Hospital-acquired infections (HAIs), also known as "nosocomial infections," are increasingly common and are challenging the commonly held view that hospitals are safe havens for healing and recovery. In fact, the most virulent, life-threatening microbes on the planet today are found in hospitals!

U.S. hospitals infect approximately 1.7 million patients each year, causing 100,000 deaths. To be absolutely clear, these are *infections contracted while visiting the hospital.*[5] In the European Union, the situation is similar: hospitals infect roughly 2 million patients and cause 175,000 deaths annually.[6] These alarming numbers are causing medical experts to question whether booking surgery in hospitals is really worth the risk. According to the WHO's Director-General, Dr. Margaret Chan: "Hospitals have become hotbeds for highly-resistant pathogens ... increasing the risk that hospitalization kills instead of cures."[7]

To add to the problem, many of the superbugs that have been confined to hospital settings for years are now becoming harder to contain. These virulent drug-resistant strains are now infecting otherwise healthy individuals in communities across the United States, Canada, and other countries.[8]

Pandemics and False Alarms

According to health authorities, a global pandemic looms on the horizon. The Spanish Flu of 1918 killed an estimated 20 to 50 million people, or one to three percent of the world's population, depending on sources. An outbreak of this magnitude today would take between 70 and 210 million lives. With rapidly evolving new drug-resistant strains emerging every year, scientists say we have every reason to think it will happen again. Many experts say it is inevitable.

But after the false alarms of the past decade, many people have become more skeptical. First it was the West Nile Virus in 2002, followed by Severe Acute Respiratory Syndrome (SARS) in 2003, Bird Flu (H5N1) in 2004, and Swine Flu (H1N1) in 2009. In each case, the media ran with it, and journalists and public health officials seemed to overplay the importance of these apparent outbreaks. After the dust settled, the number of fatalities did not support the alleged threat: 1,144 died of West Nile (U.S.),[9] 774 died of SARS; 282 died of Bird Flu,[10] and 18,000 died of Swine Flu. While tragic, these were not pandemics. To put it in perspective, the seasonal flu kills between 250,000 and 500,000 people every year.[11]

Despite all of this, health authorities continue to communicate that antimicrobial resistance is a global emergency. In her keynote address at the 2012 conference on "Combating Antimicrobial Resistance: Time For Action" in Copenhagen, Denmark, Dr. Chan stressed the urgency of the situation and the need for developed nations to wake up:

> The threat, as you have noted, is indeed global, extremely serious, and growing. ... Yet attention is still sporadic, and actions are far too inadequate. In my personal view, one problem is that the threat of antimicrobial resistance is competing for attention in a world beset by one global crisis after another.[12]

Infectious disease experts unanimously agree and all communicate the same message: It's real. Things have to change. We have to act now.

The End of the Antibiotic Era

While pathogens become increasingly drug-resistant, and the death toll from infectious disease continues to rise, another development has escalated the crisis: Pharmaceutical companies around the globe have closed their antimicrobial discovery divisions, and virtually no new antibiotics are being developed today. The retreat of industry at this critical time has been characterized as a "perfect storm."

As early as 1990, half of the large companies in the U.S. and Japan significantly reduced their antibiotic discovery efforts. Between 2002 and 2004, Bristol-Myers Squibb Company, Abbott Laboratories, Eli Lilly and Company, Wyeth, Sanofi-Aventis, Procter & Gamble, and others, either halted or substantially reduced their research and development into new antimicrobials.[13] More recently, Pfizer shut down its major antibiotic research facility in England and central lab in the U.S. In the words of Dr. Chan, "The R&D pipeline for new antimicrobials has practically run dry. ... The world is on the brink of losing these miracle cures."[14]

Scientists explain that what is needed today are new, distinctly different classes of antibiotics, for which the microbial world has no acquired defenses. From 1940 to 1968, around twenty classes of antibiotics were invented. Only three new classes have reached the market since then, and resistance to one class emerged even before the FDA approved the drug.[15] According to Chan:

> If current trends continue unabated, the future is easy to predict. Some experts say we are moving back to the pre-antibiotic era. No. This will be a post-antibiotic era. ... in effect, an end to modern medicine as we know it. Things as common as strep throat or a child's scratched knee could once again kill. Some sophisticated interventions, like hip replacements, organ transplants, cancer chemotherapy, and care of preterm infants, would become far more difficult or even too dangerous to undertake. At a time of multiple calamities in the world, we cannot allow the loss of essential antimicrobials, essential cures for many millions of people, to become the next global crisis.[16]

There are many valid reasons why antimicrobial exploration is no longer attractive to companies and their investors. Costs are exorbitant, the success rate is low, it takes years from discovery to market, sales are slow, and ultimately profit is low in relation to other drugs than can be pursued. There is a much greater financial return on drugs that patients take for life; for example, insulin for diabetes, statins for cholesterol, and drugs that treat hypertension, arthritis, impotence, and baldness. Furthermore, overuse of antibiotics accelerates their ineffectiveness and provides yet another reason why antibiotic discovery is no longer attractive. Why invest huge sums of money to develop a new antibiotic when the drug's lifespan may end before that investment is recouped? But tell this to medical and public health professionals who work on the front lines where treatments are failing, people are dying, and there is every indication that things will only be getting worse.

Despite the circumstances, health authorities hope the situation can turn around with innovative public policy. A huge effort by governments in the form of legislation, financial support and real incentives could motivate pharmaceutical companies to reinvest in this sector. Their thinking is, if enough new classes of antimicrobials could be swiftly brought to market, doctors would once again have effective treatments for infectious disease.

Natural health experts argue that unless drug companies can invent new antibiotics that don't cause resistance, what's the point? Antibiotics to date have largely failed due to their simple structures that are easily outsmarted by bacteria. We already have a solution, they say, in antimicrobial plants, which are a well-known source of complex phytochemistry that inhibits mutation and evolution of resistant strains. Unfortunately, because plants in their whole form cannot be patented, it is not profitable for drug companies, who are more inclined to seek novel inventions they can monopolize. The opinion among natural health professionals is that until the medical industry embraces whole plant chemistry, it will fail to find sustainable solutions to antimicrobial resistance.

The Real Problem: Overuse

Scientists looking for immediate solutions within the current system explain that antibiotics can serve an important role, *if and only if they are left as treatments of last resort*. Studies have shown that resistant bacteria forget how to resist antibiotics when no longer confronted with them regularly. It follows that restricting the use of antibiotics to life-threatening situations might restore and preserve the effectiveness of these drugs for years to come. Progressive countries like Sweden have demonstrated this to be true in practice, as reflected in the reduced occurrence of drug-resistant infections within their population.[17]

The real problem, they say, is not the antibiotics themselves, but the irresponsible misuse and overuse of these drugs over the past 70 years.

Antibiotics in the Environment

Each year, over *200 million pounds* of antibiotics are produced worldwide for human and animal consumption. Some estimates are twice that. This overabundance of antibacterial agents has profound consequences for humans, animals, the environment, and the many diverse species of bacteria that hold this world together.[18]

Antibiotic use creates resistant bacteria that are excreted in feces and urine into the environment, where they reproduce quickly;

one bacterium can become a billion overnight. Furthermore, this waste also contains antibiotics and their residues that remain active for months or years. In soil, streams, rivers and oceans, antibiotics continue to kill off susceptible bacteria and stimulate evolutionary development of resistant strains, which causes imbalances in our global ecosystem.

According to the late Mark Lappé, prominent toxicologist, author and educator:

> We have let our profligate use of antibiotics reshape the evolution of the microbial world... Resistance to antibiotics has spread to so many different, and such unanticipated types of bacteria, that the only fair appraisal is that we have succeeded in upsetting the balance of nature.[19]

There are many examples of how antibiotics are polluting our world. One study found different strains of drug-resistant bacteria in the eggs of sea turtles.[20] Other studies demonstrate that antibiotics and superbugs are cycling back to us in our food and water supply. There is no doubt that we live in a highly interconnected world, and our poor stewardship has caught up to us.

Antimicrobial compounds used in everyday cleaning and grooming products are another major problem. For instance, *triclosan* and *triclocarban* promote cross-resistance to many antibiotics and are proven hormone disruptors that can cause adverse developmental, reproductive, neurological, and immune effects in both humans and wildlife. Both of these chemicals are commonly found in soaps, sanitizers, shampoos, deodorants, toothpastes, mouthwashes, cosmetics, facial tissues, antiseptics, and animal grooming products. Because triclosan and triclocarban go by many different names, they are elusive, but chances are you have them in your house. In 2001, 76 percent of liquid soaps and 26 percent of bar soaps in the U.S. contained triclosan, according to research published in the *American Journal of Infection Control.*[21] To add insult to injury, studies have shown these products are no more effective at killing bacteria than scrubbing with soap and water.

Like antibiotics, these chemicals move *through* us, and travel by wastewater into the environment where they create resistant bacteria that return to us through our water, soil, and food. Research has identified both compounds in streams, surface water, aquatic sediments, and treated waste water. Their high concentration within sewage sludge is a growing concern, since this toxic sludge is commonly applied to agricultural fields as fertilizer. Logically, these chemicals find their way to the ocean too, which is especially unfortunate since triclosan is very toxic to aquatic life. A study in 2009 found the accumulation of triclosan in bottlenose dolphins, which reflects the extent to which the chemical has infiltrated the marine food chain.[22]

Meanwhile, the use of consumer products containing these chemicals is on the rise. The CDC reported in 2010 that triclosan in humans had increased by an average of 50 percent since 2004.[23] According to Richard Harth at Arizona State University's Biodesign Institute, studies have revealed that 97 percent of all U.S. women had detectable levels of triclosan in their breast milk, and 75 percent of Americans had triclosan in their urine.[24]

Dr. Sarah Janssen, Senior Scientist at the Natural Resources Defense Council, stated in a 2010 press release:

> The widespread and unregulated use of antimicrobials such as triclosan and triclocarban must end. In just two years, human exposure to triclosan has dramatically risen and now there is evidence that our food supply could also be contaminated with these chemicals. With no proven benefit and many red flags raised for harmful health impacts, the use of these so-called antimicrobials is an unnecessary and stupid use of toxic chemicals.[25]

Antibiotics in Production Animals

Of the millions of pounds of antibiotics produced each year, well more than half are used in the production of livestock and poultry. In contrast to human and veterinary medicine where treatment is directed at an individual, entire groups of healthy food animals are regularly administered antibiotics as a "growth promoter" in feed or water (sub-therapeutic dosages). The fact that more antibiotics are used in healthy animals than in unhealthy humans is a cause for great concern. Of equal concern is that most of these antibiotics are the same ones used to treat human disease, and therefore, most drug-resistant bacteria in animals also resist treatment in humans.

If we look at the United States in 2009, agriculture accounted for more than 80 percent of the 33 million pounds of antibiotics sold in the U.S., and 90 percent of that was administered sub-therapeutically through food and water.[26]

When production animals receive low doses of antibiotics daily, throughout the year, their gastrointestinal tracts become reservoirs for spreading drug-resistant bacteria into the environment. Furthermore, 30 to 60 percent of these antibiotics move *through* food animals and remain active in the environment, creating more resistant germs. Once in the soil and water, both find their way into other animals and humans. A recent study showed that cow urine continued to kill off E. coli and create resistant strains that infected nearby calves.[27]

Direct contact and eating meat are further ways in which pathogens move from animals to humans. Undercooked meat can contain antibiotic-resistant pathogens which pass to humans and pets, causing acute food-borne infections of the gastrointestinal tract (food poisoning). Though rare, these infections can lead to life-threatening neurologic, hepatic and renal conditions. Chronic disorders can also result, such as arthritis, irritable bowel syndrome, and Guillain-Barre syndrome. Food-borne illness is a serious concern today, with outbreaks on the rise and increased hospitalization and death rates.

Scientists have found that resistance can also spread by "horizontal gene transfer." This transfer occurs when bacteria freely share their genes back and forth to gain new abilities that allow them to survive environments (drugs) that threaten their survival. Meat from production animals can contain drug-resistant pathogenic bacteria *and* harmless bacteria that *both* carry antibiotic-resistant genes (ARGs). Once consumed, both types can share their genes with pathogenic bacteria residing in humans, giving them drug-resistant "powers."

Genes and Drug-Resistant Infections

Horizontal gene transfer has completely changed the way science is viewing the spread of resistance, and is believed to be the most important factor in the emergence of antibiotic-resistant pathogens. Before science understood the role of ARGs, the rise in resistant infections was believed to be caused solely by the spread of pathogens. Pathogens can be transmitted by direct contact with animals or humans, by door knobs and other places that hands frequent, and by food, soil, water and air. This *physical* spreading of germs is a serious problem, but the spread of resistance genes is more rapid and more extensive.

This is because both pathogenic and harmless bacteria can carry ARGs, and spread them quickly within entire bacterial populations of the same niche (e.g., human gut, pond, river, etc.) and across species, genus and phyla boundaries to entirely different bacterial populations.[28] Bacteria are continually sharing genes from wherever they are, *to other kinds of bacteria anywhere else*, via the world's interconnecting commensal, environmental, and pathogenic bacterial populations. This transfer of genetic coding among distantly related bacterial species and taxa helps explain why antibiotic resistance has become such a global problem. We know most of the world is made of bacteria and now science has proven that resistance "data" is being shared in every direction without limits. Scientists are calling it a massive "global network" bringing to mind how fast data travels on the internet.[29]

Antibiotic Resistant Genes in Our Food Supply

One of the lesser known issues with GMO crops and foods is that they contain antibiotic-resistant "marker genes," and some scientists are concerned about gene transfer to humans. More concerning is the possibility that non-GMO foods may also be contaminated with ARGs. One study showed that harmless and beneficial bacteria in common supermarket foods, such as seafood, dairy, deli items and fresh produce, carry genes that code for antibiotic resistance. The scientists concluded that our food supply contributes, at least partially, to the loss of antibiotic effectiveness and the continuing rise in drug-resistant infections.[30]

Antibiotic Resistant Genes in Our Environment

Not surprisingly, bacteria carrying ARGs—pathogenic, but harmless ones too—have been found throughout our environment. Hundreds of various genes encoding resistance to a broad range of antibiotics have been identified in wastewaters, sewage, surface water, groundwater, irrigation, and even in drinking water. They're in our soils too. Researchers from the Washington University School of Medicine discovered that harmless bacteria in various American soils carried the exact same ARGs found in many resistant pathogens responsible for fatal diseases (i.e., *Pseudomonas aeruginosa* and *Yersinia pestis*). How does this happen? In all likelihood, drug-resistant bacteria make their way into the environment and share their genes with soil bacteria; conversely, harmless soil microbes find their way into humans and animals where they pass along resistance genes to pathogens.

The oceans have also become reservoirs for ARGs. As with soil, marine sediment has been found to harbor the same resistance genes found in human pathogens. We can assume a similar cycle; in this case ARGs make their way back to us through the seafood we eat. Marine aquaculture contributes to the problem by using antibiotics to improve production of farmed organisms like fish and shrimp, creating drug-resistant pathogens that are free to share their genes with bacterial populations throughout the ocean.[31]

Rays of Hope

No doubt, this is a crisis that affects all citizens of the world, and all life on this planet. Stephen Harrod Buhner is a master herbalist, author, and teacher of alternative approaches to treating infectious illness. In his book, *Herbal Antibiotics: Natural Alternatives for*

Treating Drug Resistant Bacteria, Buhner states:

> We do in fact have a serious problem. We have
> meddled with the microbial world and created
> bacteria more tenacious and virulent than any
> known before. They will have effects on both
> the ecosystem and the human population that
> can only be guessed at. What is sure, however,
> is that the antibiotic era is over. The degree and
> rate of bacterial evolution is so extreme that new
> antibiotics (of which few are being developed)
> generate resistance in only a few years instead of the
> decades that it took previously. It is a frightening
> future. But there are rays of hope...[32]

"Rays of hope?" you ask. What hope could we possibly
have? We have hospitals that are infectious disease hotbeds,
superbugs in our communities, increased rates of infection-
related disease and disability, death tolls rising, a pandemic
looming, last-resort treatments failing, and every indication
that new antibiotic discovery is over. And let's be honest. We
know the pharmaceutical and agricultural industries have
a vested interest in continued massive-scale use of antibiotics.
Is there really anything we can do to turn this around?
The answer is, thankfully, a resounding "Yes!"

What We Can Do

There are a number of things each of us can do to take care of ourselves, our families and friends, and our communities:

Say "No" to Antibiotics: Don't go to the doctor and ask for an antibiotic—ask the doctor if an antibiotic is really necessary. Colds and flus are caused by viruses, not bacteria, so antibiotics are useless against them. If your doctor recommends antibiotics but isn't certain the infection is bacterial, then request that a diagnostic test be done, and wait for the results before proceeding. Newer tests are becoming available that are quick and accurate. Finally, remember that antibiotic overuse in humans contributes to drug-resistance within your community and worldwide, so do your part and find alternative ways of protecting yourself and treating infections when they arise.

Boost Your Immune System: With such prevalent use of antibiotics worldwide, you would think that they were actually safe and effective, but they are not. Antibiotics damage the immune system, your body's natural defense against infection, by killing off healthy bacteria in the gut. Science has confirmed that our intestinal flora protect us from invaders, and communicate with other parts of the immune system to ensure its correct function and health. You could safely say that our intestinal flora is our immune system. It can be the best line of defense you have, capable of fighting off the nastiest of superbugs. Therefore, take care of it. Look for natural foods, minerals, vitamins and other supplements that support your immune system. Drink lots of good water; get plenty of exercise, sleep, fresh air and natural light during the winter months; and be sure to avoid toxins—even small quantities of alcohol and cigarettes are very hard on the body.

Use Natural Alternatives to Antibiotics: When an infection arises, focus on boosting your immune system and take natural alternatives to antibiotics. Visit an herbalist, naturopath and your local health food store to discover the many natural treatments and therapies that exist.

Use Natural Alternatives to Antibacterial Products: Look at the marketplace with fresh eyes and you will notice the plethora of antibacterial products available. It's big business! Antimicrobial chemicals are found in products we might overlook, like wipes, cloths, sponges, garbage bags, cling wrap, chopping boards and even diapers and clothing. Since the pandemic scare of the past decade, companies have been preying on the fears of consumers. The fact is, these antibacterial chemicals harm your immune system and the environment, and they're unnecessary. Studies have shown that proper scrubbing of your hands with regular soap is effective at removing pathogens, without adding to the problem of antimicrobial resistance. Infectious disease experts are asking us to use good old-fashioned elbow grease to scrub away organic matter, and then questioning if disinfecting is necessary. Usually, it is not. That said, many natural products are available at your local health food store that are non-toxic and biodegradable, and disinfect without creating germ resistance. Even a simple mixture of vinegar and water is an excellent way of killing germs when you need it. A final note of caution: Be wary of big brand products in grocery and hardware stores that tout "natural," "green," or "biodegradable," as this is often false advertising. Read labels closely. You may discover that the parent company makes their bread and butter selling bleach or other chemical products. And if the ingredients are difficult to pronounce, they're probably not natural.

Mind Your Food: Raw fruit and vegetables can be covered with pesticides, antibiotics, and/or resistant germs, so soak them in a natural solution, then scrub and rinse. When it comes to meats, be sure to cook thoroughly to kill off any resistant bacteria. Furthermore, use your buying power to affect change. Especially for foods that are heavily sprayed or treated with pesticides or antibiotics, *choose organic*. Together, we may one day give producers a strong incentive to change their ways, or perhaps their line of work. Finally, be aware that in the U.S., certain varieties of organic apples and pears susceptible to fire blight are being sprayed with *streptomycin* and *tetracycline*, two antibiotics used in humans and animals. It is predicted that this will come to an end in October, 2014. Again, let your dollar speak for you; buy only those varieties that are naturally resistant to fire blight.

Educate Others: Share what you know about antimicrobial resistance and the unnecessary use of antibiotics and antibacterial chemicals. Begin with family and friends, and if the opportunity is right, reach out to people in the community. Think of it as helping others. Today, more people are awakening and appreciate hearing important truths about our world.

Demand Change: If you feel called, be an activist for change. Write your local politician expressing your concerns about the unnecessary use of pesticides, antibiotics, and chemicals in your community. Start a petition. Form a group where health and environmental concerns can be shared. Use social media to get the word out. Let your dollar speak for you; as consumers we can influence the quality and types of products in the marketplace. Organize something for Antibiotic Awareness Day on November 18th of every year. Lead by example to inspire change.

> Never doubt that a small group of thoughtful, committed citizens can change the world. Indeed, it is the only thing that ever has. - *Margaret Mead*

What They Can Do

There are a number of things our governments can do to tackle antimicrobial resistance and to protect and care for their citizens, the citizens of neighboring countries and the world. Progressive countries like Sweden and Denmark are leading the way and serve as model examples for other countries, of what works and what does not. The UN's World Health Organization has created a strategic action plan for nations to adopt, and the European Union has generated models, useful elsewhere, for combating antimicrobial resistance on multiple fronts. Australia created its own blueprint for tackling the problem, which included several recommendations in the areas of regulation, surveillance, monitoring, infection prevention, education, and research.[33]

So the point is, the first steps have been made, and today, more than ever before, there is the desire for answers, solutions, and change.

World governments need to set their sights high. This is a time for creative thinking, breaking paradigms, and taking action. Here are a few goals that most infectious disease experts, environmental scientists, health authorities and politicians can agree on:

- Restrict antibiotic use in humans and animals.
- Restrict sub-therapeutic antibiotic use in production animals.
- Restrict the use of antibiotics in aquaculture and bee farming.
- Restrict the use of antimicrobial chemicals in consumer products.
- Restrict the use of pesticides and antibiotics in fruits and vegetables.
- Implement tight regulations and enforcement on the production of man-made chemicals and technologies that may encourage bacterial resistance.
- Improve the management of waste containing antibiotic-resistant genes.
- Preserve specific drugs so they remain effective as last resort treatments.

- Explore innovative antibiotics that are safe for humans and the environment.

- Explore innovative antibiotics that are safe for animals, that are distinctly different, and that do not promote cross-resistance.

- Remove government regulations that impose restrictions on manufacturers of natural health products (NHPs) and ultimately limit consumer access to these natural medicines, *for they are safe*.

- Embrace natural medicines and alternative therapies within the current medical model, especially those that boost immunity and treat infection.

- Educate children in elementary and high schools about the antimicrobial crisis and the importance of using natural antimicrobials.

- Educate the public via web, advertising, marketing materials, and antibiotic awareness days.

Remember, *we the people* must demand it. Let us *stand up* for the microbial world, because it's our children's future.

Herbal Antibiotics

Despite all of our medical advances, science has looked at plant chemistry with renewed interest over the past 20 years. Countless studies have shown that essential oils from certain herbs possess strong antimicrobial actions, surpassing the effectiveness of leading antibiotics. In addition to their germ-killing strength, essential oils contain an unfathomable complexity of compounds that work synergistically together to ensure the survival of the plant. Because of their intricate structure, these feisty, natural compounds leave pathogens incapable of adapting and developing resistance. In contrast, antimicrobial drugs are relatively simple structures containing few chemical constituents, and this lack of complexity makes it much easier for pathogens to find ways of counteracting their effects.

Furthermore, plants and their essential oils are generally safe for human use and the environment. They are non-toxic and work in harmony with the human body, boosting the immune system with phytonutrients and restoring health with medicinal actions. And unlike their synthetic counterparts, "herbal antibiotics" are biodegradable so they do not remain active in the environment, tampering with Mother Nature's delicate balance.

Some of the better known herbal antibiotic plants include familiar names like oregano, garlic, thyme, clove, savory, cinnamon, ginger, grapefruit (seed), eucalyptus, juniper, and sage. It may be hard to believe that these plants and their essential oils could be effective at killing drug-resistant bacteria. But it is true. And not only that, some kill viral and fungal infections as well, which is something that synthetic antibiotics can't do. In fact, there are no drugs to date that can effectively eradicate viruses and cure the illnesses that they cause. Like bacteria, viruses are evading modern medicine. It is the same situation with fungi, which are notoriously difficult to kill. This is a major concern today, given that infections—bacterial, viral, and fungal—are the underlying cause of most illness and disease in North America.

With the threat of a pandemic looming and modern treatments for infection failing, public interest in essential oils is growing. And where there is funding and interest, the scientific community continues to demonstrate the antimicrobial properties of plant oils and provide validity to the claims that herbalists, aromatherapists, naturopaths and other natural health practitioners have been making for years.

Oregano Oil for Drug-Resistant Germs

Of all the essential oils that have been studied to date, oregano oil is by far the most powerful and effective against pathogenic bacteria and viruses.

Numerous studies around the world have begun to scientifically validate oregano oil's reputation for promoting health, and demonstrate its powerful infection-fighting and immune-supportive properties. In 2001, Harry G. Preuss, M.D., a professor of biophysics at Georgetown University, reported that the essential oil of oregano, at relatively low doses, was effective against *Staphylococcus aureus*. Furthermore, his research revealed that oregano oil was comparable in its germ-killing power to common antibiotic drugs, such as streptomycin, penicillin, and Vancomycin.[34] In another study, a research team at the University of Tennessee reported that oregano oil exhibited 100 percent inhibition of common drug-resistant bacteria, including *Staphylococcus aureus, E. coli, Listeria monocytogenes, Yersinia enterocolitica, Pseudomonas aeruginosa,* and *Aspergillus niger.*[35] More recently, researchers in Delhi found that oregano oil killed MRSA more effectively than 18 antibiotics it was compared against. Furthermore, it completely eradicated MRSA at a dilution of 1 to 1000.[36]

In an Australian study, 52 plant oils were tested for antibacterial and antifungal activity, and only oregano oil was considered to have "pharmacologic" action against all bacteria and yeasts tested, including *E. coli, Salmonella enterica, Pseudomonas aeruginosa, Candida albicans, Acinetobacter baumanii, Enterococcus faecalis,* and *Klebsiella pneumonia.*[37] Scientists in Scotland also found oregano oil at the top of the list, with broad-spectrum activity against all 25 different genera of bacteria tested.[38]

Another interesting fact is that the agricultural industry is looking closely at oregano oil as a safe alternative to pesticides. And the food industry has funded numerous studies exploring oregano oil as a preservative. The combination of its antibacterial strength and high antioxidant capacity has aroused great interest and substantial investment in finding ways to optimize these benefits in food while masking the taste and smell of oregano.

Used safely and successfully for over 20 years by tens of thousands of North Americans, "Oil of Oregano" has rightfully earned its reputation as a powerful infection fighter and versatile aid for a variety of ailments. Its unparalleled effectiveness against all types of pathogens, including bacteria, viruses, fungi, parasites, and protozoa, makes it useful for a wide range of infection-related conditions. Today, Oil of Oregano is being used by many naturopathic doctors and holistic vets to successfully manage conditions that would otherwise be treated with antibiotics. Dr. Kurt Schnaubelt, French-trained aromatherapist and founder of the Pacific Institute of Aromatherapy remarks, "When it comes to combating bacterial infections, oregano is aromatherapy's heavy artillery."[39]

When you consider how prevalent antibiotic-resistant infections are today, it appears that Oil of Oregano may be an answer to one of our most pressing global health concerns: How do we treat infections, now and in the future?

Infections play a much larger role in public health than we recognize, and medical doctors frequently overlook infection as the underlying cause of illness or disease. For example, a variety of diseases, such as arthritis, chronic fatigue syndrome, irritable bowel syndrome, ulcerative colitis, psoriasis, eczema, sinusitis, peptic ulcer, fibromyalgia, and gastritis—the list goes on—are frequently caused by chronic infections that are overlooked and never treated. When an infection is identified, oftentimes doctors have little to offer except antibiotics or other drugs that are known for their toxic effects on the body, and have no guarantee of working. This is why Oil of Oregano has been so well received. It is safe and effective. It can be used to treat all types of infections—from the ones you know about, to the ones you don't.

Perhaps best of all, you don't need a prescription—Oil of Oregano can be self-administered whenever an infection is suspected, or taken as a preventative to stop infection from arising.

2

Getting To Know Oregano

Not Your Average Mint

Oregano is a member of the *Lamiaceae* family of plants, commonly referred to as the "mint family." Many familiar culinary herbs are from this family, including rosemary, thyme, basil, and sage, as well as some commonly used in teas, such as peppermint, lavender, lemon balm, and catnip.

The word "oregano" comes from the Greek words *oras* ("mountain") and *ganos* ("joy"), or more simply, "joy of the mountains." Of all the species of oregano—and there are at least 40—by far the best known is *Origanum vulgare*. This particular plant is high in phytochemical compounds that fight infections and has been used repeatedly in scientific studies. However, many other *Origanum* species are equally high in these active ingredients, though they are not as well documented in Western medicine. Examples include: *O. compactum*, *O. dictamnus*, *O. hypericifolium*, *O. minutiflorum*, *O. onites*, and *O. syriacum*. All of these species, along with the better-known *O. vulgare*, are native to the higher, more mountainous regions of the Mediterranean and Middle East. Together, they are generically referred to as "Mediterranean Oregano." All species of oregano are perennial plants and can be picked wild or cultivated quite easily.

Because of this plant's strong aroma and unique flavor, oregano has long been used as an ingredient in dishes native to the Mediterranean region. However, it is important to note that most oregano available in the grocery store for culinary purposes is *not* Mediterranean oregano; it is often a variety of marjoram, a close relative of oregano, and also within the Origanum genus. Marjoram is milder and sweeter, compared to the more robust flavor of oregano. Mediterranean oregano is actually quite bitter; when picked fresh, it may even leave your tongue quite numb. It is this bitter and "hot" taste that denotes a higher amount of the active ingredients responsible for oregano's antiseptic strength, which served the Mediterranean diet well, especially before refrigeration or other sanitation methods came into use.

An Ancient Remedy

Though it is best known as a culinary herb, oregano has a very ancient medical reputation. Its oval green leaves and tubular flowers have been used for thousands of years to treat sickness, disease and injury. The Egyptians and Babylonians used oregano as far back as 3000 BC, and many scholars believe that the Biblical Hyssop was a species of Mediterranean oregano. The Greeks learned about steam distillation of plant oils from the Egyptians around 500 BC, and steam-distilled oregano oil is mentioned in medical references of that time. In Greece and Rome, oregano was revered as a powerful healing plant and was a ubiquitous symbol of joy and happiness. It was placed on graves at funerals to provide comfort and dismiss sadness, and flowering wreaths were worn by newlyweds to receive blessings of love and goodwill.

The Greek physicians Hippocrates (B.C. 460-377) and Dioscorides (A.D. 40-90) both prescribed the use of oregano for a myriad of conditions. Hippocrates used it for respiratory and gastrointestinal disorders, wounds, venomous snake and insect bites, and even hemlock poisoning! Dioscorides recommended oregano for cough and lung congestion, earache, inflamed tonsils, thrush, stomach ache, heartburn, intestinal gas, skin conditions, venomous bites, narcotic poisoning, sprains, swelling and growths, spasms, spleen disease, and jaundice. He documented these medical uses in his famous work, *De materia medica*, which would become a foundational text for future herbalists and physicians. Another Greek physician, the great Galen (A.D. 129-217) cited steam-distilled oregano oil as a "proper remedy" for lung conditions, bronchitis, and sinusitis, as well as for cough and other cold symptoms.

Throughout the Middle Ages (A.D. 500-1500), it is clear that the medicinal properties of oregano and its essential oil grew with great acclaim and spread quickly to all inhabited parts of the known world. In China, oregano was used to treat colds, fever, nausea, diarrhea, itchy skin, and jaundice. In Islamic civilizations, physicians used oregano for various infection-related diseases. In medieval England, oregano became widely used as a preservative for milk and meat. The cultivated herb and its essential oil were powerful cures for respiratory conditions, such as head colds, cough, congestion, bronchitis, pneumonia, and asthma. Digestive illnesses like diarrhea, stomach ache, intestinal worms, and food poisoning were also successfully treated. Some English herbalists also prescribed oregano for headaches, toothaches, arthritis, muscle pain, swelling, bruising, scurvy, wound healing, and disorders of the uterus, bladder, liver, and heart. The German-Swiss physician Paracelsus (A.D. 1493-1541) found it was also effective for fungal infections and psoriasis. Later in the sixteenth and seventeenth centuries, English herbalists Gerard, Langham, Culpeper, and Salmon would collectively record all of oregano's medicinal uses in their famous "herbals," which remain important traditional texts to this day.

During the colonization of the Americas, oregano became part of standard medicine. The herb was cultivated, and the steam-distilled oil became popularly known as "Oil of Oregano." In the early 1900s, American physicians were relying on this concentrated oil for its antiseptic and anti-inflammatory properties, and successfully treated all types of infections. But with the advent of allopathic medicine, traditional uses of natural remedies began to wane.

The primary aim of allopathic medicine has been to prove, irrefutably, the cause of a particular reaction in the body to a specific chemical. Though scientific, this somewhat narrow approach has made it virtually impossible for herbal remedies, including essential oils, to find their way into the halls of allopathic medicine. Every plant contains dozens, if not hundreds and even thousands, of chemical constituents that may react differently when extracted from their original source, or analyzed independently of one another.

Nevertheless, science has been able to pinpoint a few of the active properties of oregano that make it so effective.

How Does Oregano Work?

Every living plant contains natural compounds called *phytochemicals,* or plant-based chemicals. These all have different effects in our body. For example, if you eat straight ginseng you may feel a boost of energy, and your body temperature may rise slightly. This is because of the effect of a particular group of phytochemicals in ginseng called *ginsenosides* that increase adrenaline production, thus boosting energy and causing a warming effect.

In oregano, too, there are many active phytochemicals, each with its own unique properties. The phytochemical composition—and potency—of any one oregano plant is the product of various factors, such as species type, climate, growing altitude, soil conditions, and plant genetics. *Origanum vulgare* and other wild oregano species of the Mediterranean have been analyzed and shown to possess over a hundred compounds. This helps explain why oregano is so diverse in its uses and can help with so many different ailments.

Some of oregano's main constituents include *carvacrol, cymene, terpinene, thymol, limonene, pinene, isoborneol,* and *caryophyllene.* Each of these compounds serves a unique purpose, working synergistically with the others to ensure the well-being and survival of the plant.

Of these active compounds, carvacrol is the main compound responsible for oregano's renowned infection-fighting power. Essential oils containing higher concentrations of this phenolic compound have been shown to be effective in destroying pathogens (infection-causing organisms) and healing infectious illness and disease. Phenolic compounds, or "phenols," are remarkable antimicrobial compounds that are rarely found as main components within essential oils. Only a few plants are known to have a high phenolic content—notably oregano, thyme, ajowan, and some varieties of savory.

In general, wild Mediterranean oregano is known for its higher levels of carvacrol, but, in actual fact, carvacrol levels vary across different species of wild oregano. For instance, carvacrol can vary from 20 to 85 percent of essential oil content, depending on plant type and growing altitude. As a result, "Wild Mediterranean" Oil of Oregano products also vary in carvacrol potency.

> **Oregano 101:** The term "oregano oil" is commonly used to describe the pure, undiluted oregano essential oil referred to in aromatherapy texts, and used in the manufacturing of Oil of Oregano products. Over the years, "Oil of Oregano" (with capitals) has become the accepted name for marketed products containing oregano oil diluted with a carrier oil. Dilutions vary from product to product. In its pure concentrated form, oregano oil is not intended for oral or topical use, and with good reason: it is an irritant. Therefore, Oil of Oregano products are always blended with olive oil or another food-grade carrier, which also enhances the absorption of its naturally occurring phytochemicals. Carvacrol potency is the amount

of active ingredient *within the oregano essential oil* (not the diluted Oil of Oregano product) and is usually given as a percentage.

Thymol is another phenolic compound in oregano oil that has been shown in laboratory studies to work synergistically with carvacrol to boost its effectiveness. Even at low concentrations, thymol contributes significantly to oregano's overall effectiveness. This feature underscores the importance of honoring the whole plant and the innate synergy of all its compounds working together, rather than any one single ingredient. As the adage goes, the total is often greater than the sum of the individual parts!

Like other plant-derived phenols, carvacrol and thymol destroy disease-causing organisms (bacteria, viruses, fungi, parasites, and protozoa) through their membrane-active properties. They damage cell membranes or other protective outer structures to induce leakage of intracellular contents—and have proven significantly more effective (and safer) than synthetic phenol, commonly used in industrial antiseptics and insecticides. According to Dr. Schnaubelt, carvacrol and thymol are "a perfect example of the advantages natural substances hold over synthetic ones."[40]

In addition to its phenols, oregano essential oil consists of numerous terpene hydrocarbons, long-chain alcohols, and esters—all of which contribute to oregano's antimicrobial strength and complexity. Oregano is also one of the few herbs containing substantial amounts (depending upon the species) of rosmarinic acid, a potent free-radical scavenger, which helps explain oregano's powerful antioxidant action.

Carvacrol, thymol, and rosmarinic acid are just three of oregano's active compounds that have been researched in-depth and shown to have incredible medicinal value. It could be decades before researchers completely understand the actions of other compounds in the plant, and the synergistic effects of all the compounds working together.

Medicinal Properties

While we wait for science to unlock the secrets of why oregano oil has such wide-ranging health benefits, we already have a good working knowledge stemming from the French tradition of medical aromatherapy. Although the foundations of aromatherapy date back thousands of years, the actual term was not used until the early twentieth century when a French chemist by the name of René-Maurice Gattefossé became interested in essential oils for their medicinal uses. In the years following, the French model of aromatherapy was further developed by esteemed doctors Jean Valnet, Paul Belaiche, Daniel Pénoël, Pierre Franchomme, and others who relied on scientific research and empirical evidence from their practices, using whole essential oils of *therapeutic grade quality* (internally and topically). To a large extent, these pioneers of aromatherapy deserve credit for our current knowledge of oregano oil and its properties, uses, applications, and dosages. Today, oregano (origanum) can be found in most herbal and aromatherapy texts, and it is here that you will find listed the following medicinal properties...

Antibacterial, Antiviral, Antifungal, and Antiparasitic

Oregano oil is a powerful *Antimicrobial*. Numerous scientific studies and human experience have confirmed its ability to destroy many infection-causing "germs" from all five classes of pathogens: viruses, bacteria, fungi, parasites, and protozoa. When you consider how many health conditions are caused by these invading organisms, it becomes apparent why Oil of Oregano is such a useful remedy. It can be used as a preventative; for instance, to dress a wound or prevent food poisoning while travelling. Or it can be used to treat an existing infection inside or outside the body. These days, it is best known as an effective cold and flu remedy. Its powerful action against drug-resistant bacterial and viral infections makes it a suitable alternative to prescription antibiotics and other antimicrobial drugs.

Anti-inflammatory, Antispasmodic, Analgesic, Antirheumatic, and Rubefacient

Oregano oil has *Anti-inflammatory* and *Analgesic* properties, which makes it useful for many conditions where inflammation and pain are present. When applied topically, it relieves the discomfort of sore muscles and joints, athletic injuries, wounds, burns, insect bites, and other skin irritations. When taken orally, it can help with headaches and digestive discomfort. For those conditions where pain and inflammation are symptoms of infection (e.g., toothaches), Oil of Oregano is the perfect treatment; it aggressively fights the infection while relieving discomfort.

Oil of Oregano has several qualities that make it an effective topical rub for aching muscles and joints: (1) as an essential oil, it is absorbed quickly by the skin and penetrates deep into the tissue; (2) it reduces pain and soreness; (3) it reduces inflammation; (4) its *Antispasmodic* action calms spastic tissue; (5) as an *Antirheumatic*, it loosens stiff joints and improves mobility; (5) it is also a *Rubefacient*, so it increases blood circulation to the area, provides a comforting sense of warmth, and helps to clear by-products of prior inflammation; and (6) like all plant oils, it supports the body's natural repair mechanisms and healing process. With these properties, Oil of Oregano can be helpful for arthritis, back pain, sciatica, bunions, bursitis, muscle cramps, strains, and sprains. Its effects can boost even the best massage technique, and an increasing number of massage therapists are using it in their practices.

Vulnerary

As a compliment to its antimicrobial, analgesic and anti-inflammatory actions, Oil of Oregano has *Vulnerary* properties, so it speeds the healing of wounds and burns, reduces scar tissue formation, and prevents tissue degeneration. It is an invaluable item for first aid kits, and a necessity for jobsites where there is a high risk of work injury, for athletic locker rooms, for extreme sport enthusiasts, and for anyone who spends time in the backcountry.

Expectorant, Antitussive, and Febrifuge

Oregano oil is also a strong *Expectorant*, which means it loosens phlegm and mucous in the sinuses and lungs. It is also an *Antitussive* and *Febrifuge*, so it relieves coughing and combats fever. These three properties compliment oregano oil's powerful germ-fighting actions, and explain why it was historically prized as a remedy for colds, flus, and respiratory conditions like bronchitis and sinusitis.

Carminative, Choleretic, and Stomachic

Oregano oil is a *Carminative*, so it relieves gas upset and helps settle the digestive system. As a *Choleretic*, it stimulates bile excretion, which aids in fat digestion, helps keep cholesterol down, and expels toxins and waste products from your body. It is also considered a *Stomachic*, or a digestive aid and tonic, which relieves gastric disorders and improves digestion and appetite. Its anti-inflammatory and antispasmodic properties further aid digestion by relaxing and soothing spastic and inflamed tissue within the stomach and intestines. With all of these properties, Oil of Oregano is used for conditions such as indigestion, bloating, stomach cramps, nausea, diarrhea, and gas. In some cases, these are only symptoms of an underlying infection; bacteria, viruses, fungi, and parasites commonly root themselves within the digestive system and cause illness. When infection is the culprit, Oil of Oregano goes to work killing off invading pathogens, while relieving symptoms and improving digestive tract health and function.

Some medical experts recommend Oil of Oregano internally as part of a broader treatment protocol for Crohn's and colitis. These digestive conditions are often infection-related, and characterized by severe inflammation, spastic tissue, and sores. Oil of Oregano fights the infection, calms and soothes inflammation and spasms of the intestinal lining, works to heal ulcers and sores, and may help to relieve bloating and discomfort.

Tonic and Immune Stimulant

Oregano oil is considered a *Tonic*, which strengthens and enlivens the body, improves performance, and restores balance and function to body systems. It also acts as an *Immune Stimulant* by increasing the activity of white blood cells in defense against infection (*Cytophylactic*), and stimulating the liver and spleen which filter and clean the blood (*Hepatic* and *Splenetic*). As mentioned above, it also stimulates digestion and blood circulation, which indirectly supports immunity. With these properties, Oil of Oregano is an excellent choice when you are feeling sluggish and run down; it provides a boost, restores vitality, and brings balance where there is imbalance.

Nervine

Oregano oil acts as a *Nervine*, which means it strengthens and tones the nervous system, helping to restore balance and function. Many people notice a mild calming effect and report having a better night's sleep from taking Oil of Oregano. It can be helpful for anxiety, insomnia, hypertension, stress-related conditions, and other nervous disorders.

The essential oil of oregano has always provided me with amazing results in treating infectious diseases. Besides oregano oil's bactericidal action, it also prevents spasms, convulsions and nervous disorders. In my estimation, the antispasmodic qualities help to synergize its wonderful antiseptic powers, which comforts me every time I prescribe it for my patients. - *Dr. Paul Belaiche*

Other Properties

Oregano oil is a potent *Antioxidant*, so it reduces oxidative damage, which is thought to be involved in the development of many age-related diseases. In fact, it has been proven in many scientific studies to be far more effective at halting free radical production than most plants and fruits.

Herbal and aromatherapy texts also cite oregano oil as an *Antitoxic* and *Antivenom*. It counteracts the effects of toxins and poisons, and neutralizes venom from insect and snake bites. Of course, in the event of a venomous bite seek immediate medical attention. But if Oil of Oregano is frequently applied and taken orally, it will certainly help, and may keep you alive while getting to a hospital.

Buyer Beware: The Issue of Adulterated Oils

The essential oil industry has been fraught with profiteers who dilute or manipulate essential oils and then subsequently market them as "pure and natural." Although adulteration of oregano oil is relatively uncommon, it is not unheard of, and distillers can employ methods that are undetectable by laboratory analysis. As the popularity of Oil of Oregano continues to grow, both retailers and consumers will need to become more vigilant to ensure pure, high-quality products.

Adulteration of oregano oil is based upon carvacrol content, its primary active constituent. Since carvacrol levels are associated with its antimicrobial strength, there is a growing demand for oil with higher levels of this compound. Mediterranean distillers can artificially boost carvacrol content, in response to foreign businesses requesting only the highest potency oregano. One such way is by adding synthetic carvacrol. Furthermore, they may even provide a written guarantee of "pure and natural," along with laboratory analysis confirming potency.

Trusted authorities on oregano oil are established Mediterranean distillers who produce therapeutic grade essential oils for medicinal use and have long-standing reputations and decades, if not generations, of experience in the business. According to these experts, any oregano product claiming levels of carvacrol above 85 percent may be adulterated. Though a few, single oregano plants can, in fact, naturally contain higher levels of this marker compound, it requires thousands of plants to create even a small volume of oil. Quite simply, there are not enough of these plants to produce commercial volumes of oregano oil exceeding 85 percent carvacrol.

Only *genuine* oregano oil containing the plants' original, unaltered chemistry is considered safe for therapeutic use and can provide the full effectiveness and wide-ranging benefits that have made Oil of Oregano so popular in recent years.

When choosing your brand of Oil of Oregano, remember that industry experts affirm that 75 to 85 percent carvacrol is the highest natural level that can be attained, batch after batch, from the highest potency species. For products that claim more, it is "buyer beware."

3

Practical Uses for Oil of Oregano

Many books on herbs and essential oils simply tell you which plants can be used for which ailments, and provide little or no instruction on how to use them. In this book, you will learn the exact doses and how best to use Oil of Oregano for specific health issues. I hope you enjoy and also share the valuable knowledge you are about to discover. For a summary of conditions that may be treated with Oil of Oregano, see Appendix A, "List of Health Conditions."

There are many brands of Oil of Oregano to choose from. I use *Joy of the Mountains* brand, which is diluted 1:3 (25 percent pure oregano oil in a base of 75 percent olive oil) and contains unaltered, naturally-occurring carvacrol that ranges between 75 and 85 percent. In a recent Canadian study, researchers at the University of British Columbia discovered that *Joy of the Mountains* was more effective against the H1N1 virus than other Oil of Oregano brands from the Canadian marketplace claiming higher carvacrol levels and/or stronger dilutions of oregano oil to carrier oil.[41]

INTERNAL USES

Most conditions that require internal use of Oil of Oregano are infection-related and call upon Oil of Oregano's antibacterial, antiviral, antifungal, or antiparasitic action. However, for some internal conditions, other properties of Oil of Oregano may be equally valuable; specifically, its anti-inflammatory, anti-spasmodic, antitussive, carminative, choleretic, antitoxic, and/or antivenom actions, depending on the condition.

The following are general guidelines for taking Oil of Oregano internally. Dosage is based on the assumption that your Oil of Oregano comes pre-diluted at 1:3 (pure oregano oil to carrier oil), which is typical of most products on the market. Although it is pre-diluted, you will find many instances in this book where further dilution is necessary.

Caution: Products labeled "oregano oil" (as opposed to "Oil of Oregano") are pure, undiluted essential oil and require 1:3 dilution at home for safe usage (and for the directions provided herein to be applicable). For your safety and convenience, look for "Oil of Oregano" products, which are typically pre-diluted at 1:3. Since dilution can vary, check the label carefully to be sure it is adequately diluted (1:3 or more) before proceeding.

Directions

Recommended Adult Oral Dosage

For infections, take five to 10 drops. If you have never used Oil of Oregano, start with a smaller amount to see how your system tolerates it. As a preventative, take five or more drops as needed. You can take Oil of Oregano before, during, or after meals depending on your health condition and tolerance.

Frequency of Use

Three to five times per day may be sufficient depending on the individual and the particular infection. For more virulent infections, take up to 10 doses in a 24-hour period.

How to Use

Oil of Oregano is known for its "hotness." This spicy sensation is normal and dissipates quickly.

Ingestion: The easiest way to take Oil of Oregano is to place drops on the tongue and drink down with a tall glass of water.

Sublingual: A more direct route is *sublingual*, which literally means "under the tongue." Place drops under the tongue and hold for a few minutes before swallowing with water. Saliva will build quickly and the hotness will dissipate. Sublingual absorption puts oregano oil's chemistry straight into the blood where it is quickly circulated through the body, and is therefore a more direct and immediate way of treating infections. In contrast, when Oil of Oregano is swallowed (ingested) it must be processed by the digestive system before it is fully absorbed into the bloodstream. That said, ingestion of Oil of Oregano has proven to be an effective route of administration for treating all types of internal infections. Furthermore, ingestion is the preferred route for digestive conditions as it puts oregano oil's chemistry in direct contact with an upset or infected gastrointestinal tract. If you dislike the taste of Oil of Oregano, you can buy it in capsules, or if you prefer the versatility of the standard bottle with dropper, you can fill your own capsules. Oil of Oregano can also be mixed with juice, yogurt, or honey. Tomato juice is a favorite for many. Some people add small amounts to sauces, marinades, soups, salsas, dips, and salad dressings for a distinct oregano flavor and its disinfecting power that gives peace of mind when eating meats and salad greens.

Children: See "Guidelines for Children" for helpful instructions on how children should take Oil of Oregano internally, and appropriate dosages for various age groups.

Cautions

Oil of Oregano creates a spicy sensation in the mouth, which subsides. Pregnant or nursing mothers should avoid use, orally and topically. Though many pregnant and nursing women have used Oil of Oregano without any reported side effects, no safety studies have been done for women in this category. When taking the oral dosage recommended above, drink plenty of water to help flush toxins from the body. For higher doses and extended use, consider taking a probiotic supplement (see "Considerations" for more information). Use with caution if you are allergic to the Lamiaceae family of plants (basil, rosemary, thyme, mint, savory, sage, etc.). Allergic contact dermatitis and systemic allergic reaction is possible. If you experience skin rash or hives, or fast or irregular breathing, seek medical attention immediately. No known drug interactions. Keep out of the reach of young children.

Conditions & Usage

Chickenpox, Measles, and Mumps

Chickenpox, measles, and mumps are viral infections that may respond well to Oil of Oregano's natural phenolic compounds and unique phytochemistry. For all of these conditions, take the recommended oral dosage. For chickenpox and measles, also apply topically to sores that require immediate attention using a diluted mixture of 1:2 (one part Oil of Oregano to two parts olive oil). If treating facial sores, dilute at least 1:4 and avoid eyes and nostrils. For mumps, in addition to the oral dosage, apply topically to swollen glands several times per day.

Colds and Flus

There is no denying that colds and flus have become a bigger problem in recent years. Have you noticed the number of people getting sick each winter, and how outbreaks continue into the summer months? Somewhere along the line, the cold and flu season became the cold and flu *year*. And it isn't just the very young and very old that are being affected; healthy, active, young adults are also getting hit hard. Some people are getting the flu several times a year. What's going on? Natural health experts explain that people have weaker immune systems today compared to decades ago for a variety of reasons, including higher stress; increased exposure to toxins; mineral and nutritionally deficient food; poor air and water quality; use of cell phones and exposure to other electromagnetic frequencies; and the list goes on. With our natural line of defense down, it is an open door for cold and flu viruses to enter. And of course, these viruses are more virulent than ever.

Antibiotics are completely ineffective against viruses. The antiviral drugs and flu vaccines that doctors can offer are also largely ineffective. Furthermore, there is much controversy over the safety of these pharmaceuticals and the reliability of statistics that support their continued use. The truth is, modern medicine has little to offer when it comes to cold and flu viruses.

Thankfully, we have Oil of Oregano. This natural antibiotic is a safe, effective response to today's virulent cold and flu strains. Since its introduction to the market 20 years ago, it has become a popular cold and flu remedy because, quite simply, it *works*. And because its various medicinal actions make it a complete treatment, Oil of Oregano:

- Fights bacterial and viral infections.
- Boosts immunity.
- Loosens congestion in the sinuses and lungs.
- Alleviates coughing and sore throat.
- Helps with headache and fever.
- Helps protect you when others are sick.

How to Use: Take the recommended oral dosage. The sublingual route is preferred as a more direct and immediate way of treating congested and infected lungs and sinuses, and for alleviating coughing fits; however, this method is optional, and swallowing works just fine. Another way to treat a spastic cough is to apply Oil of Oregano topically to the chest. If your skin is sensitive, dilute 1:1 in additional olive oil (one part Oil of Oregano to one part olive oil). If you are suffering from a sore throat, see "Sore Throat" below. Continue the recommended oral dosage for several days after you have fully recovered and all symptoms have subsided to be sure the infection is eliminated.

Prevention: Take drops as needed. Whether at home with the kids, at the office, in the classroom, or on a plane, take Oil of Oregano with you. It provides potent protection when everyone around you is sick.

Digestive Conditions

There are many digestive conditions for which Oil of Oregano is a useful remedy. Most of these conditions are infection-related, whether bacterial, fungal, or parasitic. Many people travel with Oil of Oregano to protect themselves from food and water-borne pathogens. When food and water quality is in question, simply take several drops before and after a meal or drink.

People suffering from Crohn's and colitis have had success using Oil of Oregano as part of a broader treatment protocol. These conditions are often infection-related and characterized by severe inflammation of the intestinal lining. Oil of Oregano works to soothe and heal inflamed and damaged tissue, reduce spasms, and help with bloating, cramps, and gas—all of this, while fighting off the infectious component of the disease. However, there are many potential causes that contribute to the onset of chronic digestive disease, and individual results will vary. Due to the potential severity of these conditions, consult with a natural healthcare practitioner before trying Oil of Oregano. Begin with a few drops to see how your system tolerates it. Do not exceed the recommended oral dosage.

Indigestion, Cramping, Bloating, Gas, and Nausea

Suffering from abdominal pain, cramping, bloating, or other digestive ailments? Oil of Oregano can help. Take several drops with a tall glass of water or milk. Repeat if necessary in one to two hours. If you must eat certain foods that you know cause upset, try Oil of Oregano immediately beforehand. If your symptoms are attributed to a diagnosed infection, take the recommended oral dosage until the infection is gone. If these symptoms are frequent and regular, see a healthcare professional. If heartburn is exacerbated, discontinue use.

Lyme Disease

Lyme disease is a bacterial infection transmitted by the bite of an infected tick. In its early stages, a large rash may be seen around the area of the bite, and other rashes may appear elsewhere. Flu-like symptoms are common, including stiff neck, chills, fever, swollen lymph nodes, headaches, fatigue, muscle aches, and joint pain. As with a flu, these symptoms typically resolve within days or a few weeks. In more advanced stages of the disease, recurring attacks of painful, swollen joints are common, and neurological problems can result weeks, months, or even years after the initial tick bite. Lyme disease can be difficult to diagnose because many of its symptoms mimic those of other disorders. Of course, a tick bite is an important clue, but usually people do not recall a tick bite and are puzzled by their symptoms. If identified early, antibiotics are typically prescribed and may be helpful, but many strains are resistant. Advanced Lyme disease is notoriously difficult to cure.

Due to its proven efficacy against drug-resistant bacteria, Oil of Oregano may be helpful for this condition. Of course, for all medicines, natural and pharmaceutical alike, individual results will vary. The determining factors in success may depend on the immune health of the individual with the disease, and the commitment and consistency of treatment. A challenging aspect to Lyme disease is knowing when the infection is over and treatment can stop. The diagnostic tests typically used, called *serologies*, are criticized for being inaccurate. In a nutshell, Lyme disease is evading modern medicine. Therefore, you may decide you have nothing to lose by trying Oil of Oregano.

How to Use: Take the recommended oral dosage. During the initial stages of the disease, use Oil of Oregano topically on the bite mark and any areas where rash occurs. Use full strength from the bottle, unless treating children (see "Guidelines for Children"). Supplement the oral dosage with liberal applications to the soles of the feet, the spine, or the inside of the thighs at least two times per day (see "Internal Infections" under Topical Uses). Again, use full strength from the bottle, unless treating children. Persistent and consistent treatment is important to give Oil of Oregano a chance of success. It is also important to give your body a rest from Oil of Oregano. As a guideline, take one week off after four weeks of treatment; continue another four weeks before taking two weeks off; continue with a four-week on and two-week off cycle. It is equally important to supplement with a high-quality probiotic (see "Considerations" for more information) and lots of clean water every day to flush toxins from your body. Do not exceed six months of use without consulting with a healthcare practitioner.

Respiratory Infections and Congestion

Respiratory infections are a leading cause of death worldwide. It is estimated that pneumonia alone kills four million people annually, around 30 percent of whom are children under five years of age. Both pneumonia and bronchitis are characterized by a bad cough, lung congestion, difficulty breathing, and chest pain. Oil of Oregano is invaluable for several reasons: It fights hard against the bacteria and viruses that cause these diseases, as well as the fungi and parasites that sometimes cause pneumonia too. Furthermore, it is particularly great for relieving spastic cough, lung congestion, and inflammation and soreness of the lungs when applied topically to the chest.

How to Use: Take the recommended oral dosage. The sublingual route is preferred as a more direct and immediate way of delivering oregano oil's active compounds to the upper and lower respiratory tracts; however, this method is optional, and swallowing works just fine. Continue the recommended oral dosage for several days after you have fully recovered and all symptoms have subsided to be sure the infection is eliminated. In addition to an oral dosage, topical applications and steam inhalation are also important.

Topical Applications: Apply Oil of Oregano liberally to the chest several times per day and before bed. The oregano essential oil penetrates deeply into the chest and goes to work on infected, congested, inflamed, and spastic tissue. In addition, you can also apply Oil of Oregano to the spine and soles of the feet; this is a common method for administering essential oils in aromatherapy. Both areas absorb oregano oil rapidly into the bloodstream where it is pumped back to the heart and throughout the respiratory system. Try it and you'll be surprised at the results. Whenever you apply Oil of Oregano topically to the skin, always wait several minutes before wearing clothes to allow time for absorption. A sensation of heat and temporary redness of the skin is normal. If your skin is sensitive, dilute 1:1 in additional olive oil (one part Oil of Oregano to one part olive oil).

Steam Inhalation: Steam inhalation is an additional way of treating infected and congested lungs. Put several drops of Oil of Oregano into a bowl of steaming water. Cover your head with a large towel, close your eyes, put your face above the water (create a "steam tent"), and inhale deeply for five to 10 minutes. For lung congestion, inhale through the mouth. For nasal congestion, inhale *gently* through the nose. As a substitute, inhaling the vapors from your bottle throughout the day also helps to loosen mucus.

Whether you use one or all of the aforementioned treatments, be sure to always take the recommended oral dosage of Oil of Oregano until your respiratory infection is gone.

Sinusitis, Allergy Symptoms, and Nasal Congestion

Sinusitis and rhinitis have many possible causes and can be difficult to cure until the root cause is identified. When the condition is infection-related, Oil of Oregano can be an effective treatment, as it effectively kills off the viruses, bacteria, fungus, or molds responsible. It can also relieve inflammation and loosen congestion, which provides invaluable relief to this frustrating condition.

How to Use: Take the recommended oral dosage. The sublingual route is preferred as a more direct and immediate way of reaching the sinuses; however, this method is optional, and swallowing works just fine. In addition to an oral dosage, sinus drops are also recommended.

Sinus Drops: Oil of Oregano sinus drops are another way of loosening congestion and disinfecting the sinuses of molds, fungus, bacteria, and viruses, as well as allergens like pollen, pet dander, and dust mites. Put 10 drops in a one-ounce (30 ml) dropper bottle of organic olive oil. Shake before each use. Put two to three drops in each nostril and inhale deeply. Repeat every few hours.

Sore Throat

A sore throat is commonly experienced with the onset of a cold, but laryngitis, pharyngitis, and strep throat can also be the culprit. Strep throat accounts for over 35 percent of all cases of sore throat among children, and is caused by a bacteria called Group A Strep (*Streptococcus pyogenes*). A typical case will resolve itself within a few days, yet amazingly many doctors still prescribe penicillin or amoxicillin for this common bacterium. Because of this overprescribing, many strains have become resistant to these two antibiotics. Recent studies have shown that Oil of Oregano is highly effective against Group A streptococcal (GAS) infections. In addition to its infection-fighting power, it alleviates pain and inflammation.

How to Use: Take the recommended oral dosage. Also, make an oral rinse by putting a few drops of Oil of Oregano in a tablespoon of water. Gargle for 30 seconds, and expel. Repeat two to three times per day. Most importantly, apply Oil of Oregano liberally to both sides of the throat two or three times per day. If your skin is sensitive, dilute 1:1 in additional olive oil (one part Oil of Oregano to one part olive oil). The essential oil penetrates deeply to treat pain, inflammation, and infection. You'll be surprised at how fast your sore throat disappears!

Tooth and Gum Issues

Having trouble with periodontal disease or receding gums? Oregano oil has been found to kill many types of oral bacteria that contribute to gum disease, including *Streptococcus mutans*, which plays a major role in plaque formation, cavities, tooth decay, and bad breath. Recent studies have linked oral bacteria to heart, liver, and kidney failure, as well as bone and joint disease, so the importance of oral hygiene cannot be overstated.

How to Use: For good oral hygiene and prevention, put a couple drops of Oil of Oregano on your toothpaste, and brush your teeth as usual. Make this a daily habit for healthier teeth and gums, and to prevent cavities and avoid unnecessary dental work. Also, try rinsing your mouth in the morning and evening with a few drops of Oil of Oregano in a quarter cup (50 ml) of warm water. For oral infections, such as cavities and abscesses, soak a Q-Tip or cotton swab in Oil of Oregano and apply directly to the infected or inflamed area as frequently as needed to alleviate inflammation and pain. Alternatively, put a drop or two on a clean finger and apply. Also use the oral rinse (mentioned above) several times per day.

TOPICAL USES

The following are general guidelines for using Oil of Oregano externally. More specific directions for various conditions follow, and are given with the assumption that your Oil of Oregano comes pre-diluted at 1:3 (pure oregano oil to carrier oil), which is typical of most products on the market. Although it is pre-diluted, you will find many instances in this book where further dilution is necessary.

Caution: Products labeled "oregano oil" (as opposed to "Oil of Oregano") are pure, undiluted essential oil and require 1:3 dilution at home for safe usage (and for the directions provided herein to be applicable).

> For your safety and convenience, look for "Oil
> of Oregano" products, which are typically pre-
> diluted at 1:3. Since dilution can vary, check the
> label carefully to be sure it is adequately diluted
> (1:3 or more) before proceeding.

Oil of Oregano is used topically for one of three reasons: (1)
to treat an internal infection; (2) to treat a topical infection;
or (3) for external conditions that are not infection-related,
whether it be injury, disease or first aid emergency.

Internal Infections: Many infection-related conditions for
which an oral dosage is recommended also benefit from topical
applications (for examples, see specific conditions under
"Internal Uses"). Topical applications can be used alone, but
are more commonly used in conjunction with an oral dosage.
This increases the total amount of active ingredient at work in
the body, and provides a different angle of attack; using a variety
of approaches can make all the difference in the battle against
today's virulent infections. With children, topical applications
for internal infections are often preferred, due to the taste of
Oil of Oregano. For those younger than four years, it is the
only recommended route of administration (see "Guidelines
for Children").

Topical Infections: Topical applications of Oil of Oregano are
more commonly used to treat topical infections. Depending
on the type or severity of infection, an oral dosage may also
be recommended. Examples are an acute wound infection, a
dog bite, or chickenpox.

External Conditions (no infection): There are also many external conditions that are not infection-related, that respond tremendously to Oil of Oregano's many other medicinal properties. Treatment of these conditions is always limited to topical applications directly on the affected areas. This differs from topical applications for internal infections, which are typically applied to the soles of the feet or spine, or the skin closest to an infected organ.

Directions

How to Use

For treatment of internal infections: In addition to the recommended oral dosage, you may also wish to apply Oil of Oregano liberally to the soles of the feet or along the spine. These areas are very absorptive; oregano oil's active chemicals quickly pass through the skin and into the bloodstream, circulating through the body to fight infections wherever they lie. To treat an infected organ, Oil of Oregano may also be applied to the skin closest to that organ (e.g., lungs, kidney, bladder, urinary tract, stomach, intestines, etc.). Wait several minutes before wearing clothes to allow time for absorption.

For treatment of topical infections and external conditions: Apply Oil of Oregano liberally to the infected or affected area using a clean hand or finger. Depending on skin sensitivity and the specific condition being treated, it may be necessary to dilute Oil of Oregano with additional olive oil, up to a 1:4 ratio.

Children: See "Guidelines for Children" for directions on how to prepare and use Oil of Oregano topically on children of various ages.

Frequency of Use

Unless otherwise specified for a specific condition (below), repeat several times per day and reapply before bed.

Cautions

Heat sensation and temporary skin redness is normal. Oil of Oregano may irritate sensitive skin. Dilute in olive oil according to skin sensitivity and specific condition (below). Dilute for nostrils and genital mucosae. Avoid eyes. Avoid ear canals unless well diluted (see "Ear Infections"). To remove Oil of Oregano from eyes, flush thoroughly with water. Pregnant or nursing mothers should avoid use, orally and topically. Though many pregnant and nursing women have used Oil of Oregano without any reported side effects, no safety studies have been done for women in this category. Use with caution if you are allergic to the Lamiaceae family of plants (basil, rosemary, thyme, mint, savory, sage, etc.). Allergic contact dermatitis and systemic allergic reaction are possible. If you experience skin rash or hives, or fast or irregular breathing, seek medical attention immediately. No known drug interactions. Keep out of the reach of young children.

Conditions & Usage

Acne Pimples and Clogged Pores

Rub a single drop gently on each pimple before bed. Facial skin is sensitive and requires further dilution when covering larger areas to avoid excessive irritation and redness. If your face has a number of pimples in close proximity requiring several drops, dilute 1:2 (one part Oil of Oregano to two parts olive oil) or up to 1:4. For pimples and acne elsewhere on the body, use directly from the bottle or dilute 1:1 for sensitive skin. Avoid eyes and nostrils. A mild heat sensation and redness is normal and will subside.

Cold Sores

Many people suffer through painful outbreaks of cold sores. They need suffer no more! Oil of Oregano has been used effectively as a potent antiviral, and many people swear by it for this particular condition. When the tingling sensation of an outbreak begins, apply one or two drops to the affected area several times throughout the day until the sore has gone.

Cuts, Wounds, Blisters, Bruises, and Burns

One reason why Oil of Oregano has been touted as "A Medicine Chest In A Bottle" is its ability to effectively treat cuts, scrapes, blisters, burns, and wounds of all types including surgical wounds. Add to this list bruising and swelling caused by injury, and what you have is a remedy that no first aid kit should be without. Oil of Oregano acts as a powerful disinfectant that penetrates deeply into damaged tissue to fight infection wherever it lies. It also reduces inflammation and pain associated with burns, blunt injuries, and more common "owies." And for all types of tissue damage, Oil of Oregano rapidly speeds healing so that tissue regenerates quickly, free of infection, and with minimal scar tissue. Many people have used Oil of Oregano successfully on hospital wounds that are at high risk of drug-resistant infection. These large incisions lined with stitches typically leave unsightly battle scars, but regular applications of Oil of Oregano keep scar tissue to a minimum, and often doctors are amazed at the rate and quality of healing. And for those who bruise easily, or dislike the unsightly appearance of painful contusions, Oil of Oregano's phytochemicals quickly reduce swelling and discomfort, speed healing of damaged capillaries, and make bruises smaller and less noticeable.

How to Use: If an infection already exists, apply liberally to the affected area several times per day and take the recommended oral dosage. To disinfect, speed healing, and reduce pain, inflammation and bruising, apply liberally to the affected area several times per day. As an antiseptic, Oil of Oregano may cause an initial stinging sensation, depending on the condition, but within a few minutes the analgesic properties of the oil will reduce any discomfort.

Caution: Seek medical attention if needed. Do not apply Oil of Oregano to burnt facial skin unless it is very well diluted (at least 1:4). Facial skin is often too sensitive for direct application.

Dandruff

Add several drops to a handful of shampoo, and mix before applying to head. Work into your scalp and wait five minutes before rinsing. Avoid eyes.

Ear Infections

Ear infections are one of the most common reasons parents take their children to the doctor. When used correctly, Oil of Oregano is an ideal treatment. It fights the viruses and bacteria causing ear infections, and helps relieve pain and inflammation.

How to Use: Take the recommended oral dosage (for children, see "Guidelines For Children"). Apply Oil of Oregano liberally around the ear several times per day. Diluted ear drops may also be helpful, but read the "Caution" section below before proceeding. Start by putting 10 drops in a one-ounce (30 ml) dropper bottle of organic olive oil. This strength is comfortable for most people. If you find it too strong, you can always dilute the mixture in the ear canal by adding pure olive oil to reduce the strength and flush it out. Run warm water over the bottle to warm the mixture before use. Lying on your side, squeeze several drops into the infected ear. Wait for several minutes or as long as you are comfortable. When you arise, have a tissue handy to wipe up the drops; alternatively, plug your ear with some cotton to keep the oil inside longer and allow more time for the Oil of Oregano to do its work. Ear drops can be used at your own discretion, but once or twice per day is enough, in conjunction with an oral dosage and topical applications.

Caution: Do not use ear drops if you have ear tubes, are experiencing discharge, or have reason to think the ear pain may be attributed to something other than an infection. In these cases, consult a healthcare professional and get an ear examination.

Genital Region

For herpes outbreaks, dilute Oil of Oregano in more olive oil (up to a 1:4 ratio). Apply a single drop to each sore, and allow time for absorption. Try a few drops on a Band-Aid to prevent the oil from spreading or being absorbed by underwear. For burning and itching associated with yeast infections, dilute 1:4 (one part Oil of Oregano to four parts olive oil) and apply to the genital region. As a general rule, avoid the anus and genital mucous membranes; however, if it is well diluted, oregano oil can be applied to these areas without too much discomfort. If you need to remove Oil of Oregano quickly, use a tissue or cotton pad soaked in tea tree oil to wipe off. Tea tree oil is a handy item to have available for this reason.

Hand and Foot Warts

Soak skin in hot water for five minutes and then dry. Remove dead skin using an emery board or pumice stone. Apply a drop to the wart and allow time for absorption. Repeat several times per day. Alternatively, try several drops on a Band-Aid, or soak a thin cotton pad and use tape to secure tight. Warts are stubborn, so only persistent treatment will give Oil of Oregano a chance to work.

Hand Disinfectant

With our increasing population, rapid rise in the use of hand-held devices, and frequent visits to public buildings, public restrooms, gyms, schools, and crowded offices, washing your hands regularly is more important than ever. Oil of Oregano is a powerful hand disinfectant that can be added to soap, or used alone as a hand sanitizer. And it is safe for the environment!

How to Use: Add a few drops of Oil of Oregano to your soap bar to counteract the many antibiotic-resistant strains of bacteria floating around in the world today. Oil of Oregano will boost the germicidal power of your soap to help properly disinfect your hands. If you have a soap pump at home or in the office, mix a few drops of Oil of Oregano in with your liquid soap. Have a bottle handy in your car, purse, and office to use after opening doors and shaking hands. Simply rub several drops between both hands as you would any hand sanitizer. The germicidal effectiveness of Oil of Oregano is unmatched.

Head Lice

If you experience persistent itching, feel a tickling sensation, or see small white spots stuck to your hair, you may have head lice.

There are many common treatments for head lice available from your pharmacy or doctor, but did you know that many such treatments contain harmful chemicals which have been linked to eczema and other skin conditions, and even cancer? Many people report inflammation and swelling of the scalp, and even mood swings, when using these chemical-based treatments. Oil of Oregano is a safer and more effective treatment for head lice.

How to Use: Dilute Oil of Oregano 1:2 in olive oil (one part Oil of Oregano to two parts olive oil). Massage a generous amount of diluted oil into your scalp and hair. Avoid eyes. Leave in for an hour or longer, and then shampoo and rinse. Repeat if needed until the problem is gone. Alternatively, place 20 drops of Oil of Oregano into a 200 ml spray bottle and fill up the rest with warm water. Spray your scalp three or four times per day with this solution, and in two or three days the head lice will be gone. Remember to avoid the eyes.

Nail Fungus

Apply Oil of Oregano frequently to the infected area, ensuring it gets around and underneath the nail. Try soaking a thin cotton pad with the oil, and use adhesive tape to secure the pad against your nail. Experiment with a finger cot to contain the oil around the nail bed and prevent it from spreading to keyboards, clothing, linens, and the like. Nail fungus is a virulent infection that requires regular and persistent treatment.

Scabies

Prescription treatments for scabies are known for being toxic. Oil of Oregano is a natural antiparasitic that many people have successfully used for this condition. Dilute Oil of Oregano 1:2 in olive oil (one part Oil of Oregano to two parts olive oil). Apply it evenly from your neck down to your toes, lightly coating every square inch of your body, and being careful to avoid mucous membranes (genitals, anus, eyes, and nostrils). Apply Oil of Oregano full strength to visibly infected areas, depending on individual skin sensitivity. For men with thick body hair, it is recommended that you trim hair short. This will reduce the amount of oil required to cover your body and help ensure that it is spread evenly to all areas. Allow time for absorption before wearing loose clothing. Wash and rinse after 12 hours. Follow normal procedures for cleaning linens, carpets, furniture, and clothing. Reapply Oil of Oregano to visibly infected areas in the days to follow.

Caution: Do not use this treatment if you suspect you are pregnant or nursing, or if you suspect you may have an allergy to Oil of Oregano.

Skin Conditions

One of the reasons Oil of Oregano has become so popular in recent years is its versatility in treating a wide range of skin conditions. Once again, this is due to an extraordinary combination of medicinal actions that work together to make Oil of Oregano a complete treatment. Use it to treat topical viral, bacterial, fungal and parasitic infections, and any external conditions that exhibit inflammation, swelling, pain, irritation, dryness, itchiness, and slow healing. Examples of skin conditions not already mentioned in other sections of the book are: ringworm, rosacea, shingles, herpes outbreaks, athlete's foot, stinging nettle, psoriasis and eczema, insect bites, sores, rashes, boils, and dry and cracked skin.

How to Use: Some skin conditions stem from internal infections that require an oral dosage and topical applications several times per day. Examples are ringworm, rosacea, and herpes outbreaks.

Other skin conditions are localized, topical infections that require applications to the skin only, several times per day. And then there are external conditions that benefit from oregano's other medicinal actions, where topical application several times per day is all that is required. For more information, see information directly under "Topical Uses." Psoriasis and eczema may benefit from topical applications of Oil of Oregano; however, infection is only one of many potential causes for these conditions and it is best to seek the advice of a holistic practitioner.

Sore, Injured, or Spastic Muscles

Many people find that topical application of Oil of Oregano helps with sore and spastic muscles and more severe athletic injuries. An increasing number of massage therapists are using Oil of Oregano in their practice and recommend it to their clients.

Oil of Oregano has several qualities that make it an effective topical rub for aching muscles and joints: (1) as an essential oil, it deeply penetrates tissue and reaches the source of the problem; (2) it reduces pain; (3) its anti-inflammatory action pairs well with its antispasmodic action to relax and sooth inflamed and spastic tissue; (4) it is also an antirheumatic, which means it eases the stiffness of joints and improves mobility; and (5) like all plant oils, it supports the body's natural repair mechanisms and healing process.

How to Use: Apply Oil of Oregano liberally and massage into your skin. If you are covering a larger area, you may want to dilute the Oil of Oregano in more olive oil (1:1 ratio) to make your bottle last longer.

Sore Joints

Whether your joint problems are chronic or caused by a new injury, Oil of Oregano helps. Apply liberally and massage the oil into the joint from all sides, several times per day. Many people suffering from arthritis swear by it.

Sunburns

Oil of Oregano is an effective treatment for sunburn as it reduces inflammation, prevents blistering, and speeds healing by helping cells rejuvenate faster. It quickly turns mild sunburns into a tan.

How to Use: Mix a few drops of Oil of Oregano into a tablespoon of aloe vera gel, and apply immediately after sun exposure to ease burning or inflammation and prevent blistering. Reapply as needed over the next few days to assist healing and prevent skin from peeling. As an antiseptic, Oil of Oregano causes an initial stinging sensation, but within a few minutes the analgesic properties of the oil will reduce any discomfort.

Caution: Do not apply Oil of Oregano to burnt facial skin unless well diluted (at least 1:4). Burnt facial skin is too sensitive for direct application.

GUIDELINES FOR CHILDREN

The following are general guidelines for using Oil of Oregano with children. Dosage and directions are based on the assumption that your Oil of Oregano comes pre-diluted at 1:3 (pure oregano oil to carrier oil), which is typical of most products on the market. Although it is pre-diluted, Oil of Oregano requires further dilution for topical application to younger children (see below).

Mixing the correct dilution for your child's age is a starting point; you will then find directions for specific conditions in this book that ask you to dilute your mixture even further.

Caution: Products labeled "oregano oil" (as opposed to "Oil of Oregano") are pure, undiluted essential oil and require 1:3 dilution at home for safe usage (and for the directions provided in this book to be applicable). For your safety and convenience, look for "Oil of Oregano" products, which are typically pre-diluted at 1:3. Since dilution can vary, check the label carefully to be sure it is adequately diluted (1:3 or more) before proceeding.

Internal Use

Most conditions that require internal use are infection-related and call upon Oil of Oregano's antibacterial, antiviral, antifungal, or antiparasitic action. However, for some internal conditions, other properties of Oil of Oregano may be equally valuable; specifically, its anti-inflammatory, anti-spasmodic, antitussive, carminative, choleretic, antitoxic, and/or antivenom actions, depending on the condition.

Recommended Oral Dosage

Do not give Oil of Oregano orally to children under four years of age. For children aged four to nine years, use three drops, three to five times per day. For children 10 and older, use five drops, three to five times per day.

How to Use

Oil of Oregano is known for its "hotness." This spicy sensation is normal and dissipates quickly. The easiest way to take Oil of Oregano is to place drops on the tongue and drink down with a tall glass of water or juice. Do not put drops in your child's mouth without having the drink ready, and first giving him/her clear instructions on the importance of drinking down the entire glass.

Many children dislike the taste of Oil of Oregano. You can try mixing the drops in juice, yogurt, or honey. You can also buy Oil of Oregano capsules, or if you prefer the versatility of the standard bottle with dropper, you can fill your own capsules. As another alternative (or in addition to an oral dosage), Oil of Oregano can be applied topically to treat internal infections. However, some conditions are best treated orally (e.g., digestive complaints).

Do Not Use

Children under four years of age should not take internally. See "Cautions For Children" below.

Topical Use for Internal Infections

Oil of Oregano can be applied topically to treat all types of internal infections (colds, flus, measles, mumps, etc.). Given its bitter and hot taste, this can be a nice alternative to an oral dosage. For children under four, it is the only recommended route of administration.

How to Prepare

Dilute Oil of Oregano in additional olive oil, according to age and skin sensitivity. For children aged six months to three years, dilute Oil of Oregano at a 1:4 ratio. For children four or older, dilute 1:1 or 1:2. For children 10 and older, applying the oil directly from the bottle is usually fine.

How to Use

Apply several drops to the soles of the feet or along the spine. These areas are very absorptive; Oil of Oregano quickly passes through the skin and into the bloodstream, and circulates through the body to fight infections wherever they lie. To treat an infected organ, apply several drops to the skin closest to that organ (e.g., lungs, kidney, bladder, urinary tract, stomach, intestines, etc.). Wait several minutes before wearing clothes to allow the essential oil time to absorb into the skin. A sensation of heat and temporary redness of the skin is normal.

Frequency of Use

Unless otherwise specified, apply oil several times per day and reapply before bed (see frequency of use recommendations for various conditions under "Topical Uses" in the adult section).

Do Not Use

Do not use with infants under six months of age. See "Cautions For Children" below.

Topical Use for External Conditions

Oil of Oregano can also be applied topically for all manner of bacterial, viral, fungal, and parasitic infections that manifest externally on the body. Examples include infected wounds, cuts and sores, rashes, measles, chicken pox, scabies, lice, acne pimples, and cold sores. Many other external conditions, not infection-related, benefit from Oil of Oregano's anti-inflammatory, pain-killing, vulnerary, expectorant, antitussive, and other medicinal properties. Examples are bee stings, bumps and bruises, strains and sprains, wounds, congestion, cough, and allergy symptoms.

How to Prepare

Dilute Oil of Oregano in additional olive oil, according to age and skin sensitivity. For children aged six months to three years, dilute Oil of Oregano at a 1:4 ratio. For children four or older, dilute 1:1 or 1:2. For children 10 and older, applying the oil directly from the bottle is usually fine.

How to Use

Apply several drops topically to the infected or affected area, using a clean hand or finger. Wait several minutes before wearing clothes to allow the essential oil time to absorb into the skin. A sensation of heat and temporary redness of the skin is normal.

Frequency of Use

Unless otherwise specified, repeat several times per day and reapply before bed (see frequency of use recommendations for various conditions under "Topical Uses" in the adult section).

Do Not Use

Do not use with infants under six months of age. See "Cautions For Children" below.

Cautions For Children

Children under four years of age should not take internally. Infants under six months of age should not be given topical applications. Though many parents have administered Oil of

Oregano to children under these ages, both orally and topically, without any reported side effects, no safety studies have been done.

When taking the oral dosage recommended above, drink plenty of water. For higher doses and extended use, consider taking a probiotic supplement (see "Considerations" for more information). When used topically, heat sensation and temporary skin redness is normal. Dilute in olive oil according to skin sensitivity. Avoid eyes, ear canals, nostrils, and genitals. Children should avoid touching Oil of Oregano with their hands, as it will inevitably end up in their eyes. Please educate your child about this matter. To remove Oil of Oregano from eyes, flush thoroughly with water. Keep out of the reach of young children. No known drug interactions.

Use with caution if your child is allergic to the Lamiaceae family of plants (basil, rosemary, thyme, mint, savory, sage, etc.). Allergic contact dermatitis and systemic allergic reaction are rare, but possible. If your child experiences skin rash or hives, or fast or irregular breathing, seek medical attention immediately. Consider doing a test on a small area of skin before using larger amounts on larger areas.

HOUSEHOLD USES

Fruit and Vegetable Wash

How many times have we heard in the news about people getting *hepatitis* A from strawberries grown in Mexico, or *Salmonella* or *E. coli* food-poisoning from California-grown spinach or sprouts? Who knows where your store-bought fruits and veggies have been, or whose hands they have been in contact with. Oil of Oregano can be used as an excellent fruit and vegetable disinfectant to kill food-borne pathogens in your salads and other raw foods.

Let's not forget that fruits and vegetables from the grocery store that are not "certified organic" contain herbicides and pesticides. These chemicals accumulate in our system and are linked to devastating, life-long diseases and deformities in children and unborn fetuses. Since they are oil-based, herbicides and pesticides will not come off by rinsing alone. Oil of Oregano's compounds can help remove these harmful chemical residues as well.

How to Use: In a sink or a glass bowl, add 10 drops of Oil of Oregano to a small amount of natural dish soap or fruit and veggie wash, but be sure it is 100 percent plant-based. Fill a basin with warm water, and stir until suds form. Add the fruits or vegetables, and let them sit for about 15 minutes. After soaking, use a soft veggie brush to scrub the produce. For best results, add a drop of Oil of Oregano directly to your scrub brush. Rinse well. For delicate items like strawberries and spinach, soak in the sink or bowl for 15 minutes, and then rinse thoroughly in warm water before allowing to dry. Be sure to clean your container or sink because it will now be soiled with chemical residues from your produce.

Household Disinfectant

Have you ever wondered what makes things smell the way they do? Many pleasant smells are due to active phytochemicals in the plants that surround us. Many unpleasant smells come from pollution and synthetic chemicals in the environment, and some particularly repulsive smells come from bacteria. Scientific research is showing that an alarming number of germs and bacteria are present in the air we breathe. Luckily, there is an effective way to not only eliminate foul odors but also prevent the spread of illness in your home, office, or community.

Oregano essential oil is extremely volatile, meaning it evaporates easily. As a result, it can be used in a common household diffuser to completely eliminate odors and disinfect the air. When a family member is sick, diffusing Oil of Oregano's phytochemicals into the air not only helps the sick one but also helps prevent others from catching the bug. Oil of Oregano is safe to diffuse throughout the year to keep your environment germ and odor-free.

There are a number of different types of diffusers on the market. Candle-type diffusers are the most common, but ultrasonic diffusers and nebulizers are better options, if your budget permits.

How to Use

Air: If you have a diffuser, follow the directions for your specific model and use Oil of Oregano as the diffusing oil. If you do not have a diffuser, put 100 drops in a clean 500 ml spray bottle full of water and shake well before each use. With this low-cost approach, you can mist the air in your home, as well as your carpets and furniture.

Countertops/Bathrooms: Routinely spraying your countertops with a dilution of Oil of Oregano will help keep your environment germ-free. Because Oil of Oregano is non-toxic, it will not pollute your home or the environment with harmful chemicals. Nor will it promote resistant strains of bacteria. Add a minimum of 100 drops of Oil of Oregano into a 500 ml spray bottle of water, shake well, and spray away. Be sure to shake the spray bottle well before each use.

Carpet: With the same ratio (100 drops to 500 ml) in a spray bottle, lightly spray your carpets before vacuuming for a nice, refreshing scent. This technique helps eliminate carpet mildew and mold, as well as any bugs that may be lurking in the carpet from your pets. Be sure to shake the spray bottle well before each use.

Note: Pure undiluted oregano oil can be used instead of Oil of Oregano for the applications mentioned above, mixed at a ratio of 25 drops to 500 ml of water.

Did You Know? Some hospitals in France and England are diffusing oregano oil and other essential oils to eliminate air-borne pathogens. And in Japan, some companies are using oregano oil in the air-conditioning systems to help reduce employee sickness and improve mood and productivity.

Plant Protection

Oil of Oregano can be used to treat many types of plant diseases and eliminate pests, because it contains all of the phytochemicals that protect the oregano plant from bugs and pathogens in nature. One of the many phytochemicals found in Oil of Oregano is called *limonene*. Limonene helps protect oregano leaves in the wild from insects and other pests by mimicking an insect hormone that repels other insects. Other phytochemicals found in oregano oil fall into a category called *terpenoids*, which kill molds and other forms of fungi.

How to Use: Start with 25 drops of Oil of Oregano in a 500 ml spray bottle of water. Shake well before each use. Spray the area of concern, or the entire plant in the case of insects. Be sure to spray under the leaves as well. Avoid spraying plants in direct sunlight to prevent "burning" of leaves; for best results, wait until the end of the day. Repeat every day, and discontinue treatment when plant health is restored and/or pests are gone. Often pests originate in plant soil. In addition to spraying the plant (above), use a water mixture to kill all stages of pests that may be present in the soil. Mix 25 drops of Oil of Oregano into 500 ml of water and pour around the base of the plant during typical watering times. After watering, spray the surface of the soil with a more concentrated mixture of 100 drops per 500 ml to kill any insects that may come to the surface after watering.

4

Pets and Oil of Oregano

Pet owners will be pleased to learn that Oil of Oregano can help cut down on expensive visits to the vet for many common ailments. Veterinarians may prescribe antibiotics for certain conditions, but be aware they are increasingly ineffective due to the resistant strains of bacteria commonly shared between humans and pets. It is for this reason that Oil of Oregano should be included in any protocol, whether it is used as a sole treatment or in combination with antibiotics. Whenever antibiotics are used, be sure to follow up with probiotics to replenish healthy intestinal bacteria.

It is important to select a brand of Oil of Oregano that has preparations made specifically for dogs and cats, with dosages given by weight. Some brands, like *OregaPet*, feature an entire pet line including natural first aid formulas, natural flea treatments, ear drops, oral drops, and dental sprays. Adding Oil of Oregano to a pet's daily feeding regimen can provide excellent "insurance" for your pet's overall health and wellness.

Internal Use

Many veterinarians believe that a healthy digestive system is a key foundation for a healthy animal, maximizing the potential for a long, disease-free life. Use Oil of Oregano regularly to support your pet's digestive system and keep them free of parasites and other infections.

Signs of an intestinal infection may include: diarrhea, vomiting, changes in breathing, coughing, seizures, fever, nosebleed, nasal discharge, weight loss, fatigue, scooting, irregular stool, swollen abdomen, gas, hair loss, rash, itching, matted fur, growths, local swelling, bumps, constipation, dandruff, oily coat, or rancid odor.

Always consult your veterinarian first to determine the cause of your pet's symptoms. If an intestinal infection is confirmed, Oil of Oregano may be all that is required to eliminate it.

How to Use: Use pet-strength Oil of Oregano drops as directed.

Ear Infections

Ear infections are among the most common reasons for a visit to the vet. Dogs are far more prone to ear problems than cats. Signs of ear infection include ear scratching, red ear canals, head shaking, strong odor, dark granules, and/or loss of balance. In cases of deep ear blockage, fluid discharge, or ruptured ear drum, consult a veterinarian.

How to Use: Use pet-strength Oil of Oregano ear drops as directed.

Dental Health

Dental disease among pets is skyrocketing, with up to 80 percent of pets over three years old having some degree of dental disease. Good dental health can actually prolong your pet's life by preventing other health problems from arising.

The primary culprit in dental disease is *Streptococcus mutans*, the main bacteria involved in plaque formation in both people and pets. Once the bacteria attaches to the tooth surface, it begins to attract other bacteria, which eventually forms dental plaque. These bacteria release acids that break down tooth enamel and cause cavities, bad breath, and tooth rot. As the plaque builds up, it may also cause infection of the gums, or "gingivitis," which can progress into a more serious form of gum disease known as periodontitis. At this point, bacteria and their by-products may enter the pet's bloodstream and lead to heart, liver, and kidney problems, as well as bone and joint disease.

The key to prevention is to destroy the bacteria with Oil of Oregano *before* it attaches to the tooth's surface. Pet-specific products containing oregano oil, including mouth drops, toothpaste, dental spray or treats, are available for this purpose. Also use Oil of Oregano internally to help fight against systemic infections in the bloodstream and other organs.

Watch for signs of dental problems in your pet, such as bad breath, tartar, missing or damaged teeth, inflamed or bleeding gums, excessive drool, gagging, slow eating, or eating with a tilted head. More serious cases of dental disease require a more multi-faceted approach to effectively disinfect, stabilize, and manage your pet's oral health moving forward.

How to Use: Use pet-strength Oil of Oregano toothpaste, dental spray, dental treats, or drops as directed.

Topical Use

Oil of Oregano speeds wound healing and is an excellent treatment for all types of bacterial, fungal, and parasitic infections. Use topically on ringworm, mites and insect bites, rashes, burns, hotspots, abscesses, boils, minor cuts, scratches, and stings.

Oregano oil can also be sprayed directly on your pet and its bed as a defense against fleas, ticks, mites, lice, fungal/viral/bacterial infection, ringworm, chiggers, mosquitoes, sand flies, itching, mange, and parasitic infection. You can also use it to deodorize litter boxes, dog houses, and pet caddies.

How to Use: Use pet-strength Oil of Oregano topically as directed. Use pet-strength Oil of Oregano spray as directed.

MRSA Infections

MRSA infection can be fatal for both humans and pets, and recent reports indicate it is on the rise in cats and dogs. Overuse of antibiotics has been blamed for this increase, as well as for the rise of other resistant strains of bacteria. Drug treatment for MRSA is not only expensive but also potentially harmful for pets.

Oil of Oregano helps your pet fight back against MRSA infection, both externally and internally. Keeping any wounds or skin irritations clean and disinfected with an Oil of Oregano gel is of primary importance, while Oil of Oregano drops taken orally offer an excellent way to combat the infection from the inside. Scientists in Delhi found that oregano oil killed MRSA more effectively than 18 antibiotics it was compared against. Furthermore, it completely eradicated MRSA at a dilution of 1 to 1000.[42]

Salmonella Poisoning

Are you keeping pets (and children) safe from Salmonella? Salmonella food poisoning causes severe sickness and over 600 deaths each year in North America. Five-year-old children are five times more likely than adults to contract Salmonella poisoning. Investigators believe this may be due to contact with pets that are infected with Salmonella from contaminated food and smoked treats. Protect your pet with Oil of Oregano to help reduce risk of infection.

How to Use: Use pet-strength Oil of Oregano drops as directed.

Cats, Oregano Oil, and Phenols

There is some confusion about the safety of giving cats Oil of Oregano, due in part to a misunderstanding about the nature of the phenols found in the oil.

Oil of Oregano contains the naturally occurring "monoterpene" phenols, carvacrol and thymol. These natural phenols are related to the beneficial antioxidant "polyphenols," found in fruits, berries, vegetables, green tea, red wine, and honey. Like other plant-derived phenols, carvacrol and thymol destroy microbes by damaging their cell membranes or other protective structures. Catnip, for example, also contains natural phenols. The natural phenols found in oregano oil are safe for cats, at proper dosages.

However, synthetic or "artificial" phenols should always be avoided. They can cause phenol poisoning in all mammals, especially cats because they lack the liver enzymes necessary to break down these toxic compounds. Synthetic phenols are found in gasoline, motor oil, soaps, fertilizers, paints, adhesives, drugs, vaccines, shampoo, pesticides, herbicides, and a host of other common products.

Comparing synthetic phenols and natural phenols is like comparing motor oil to olive oil. According to Dr. Schnaubelt, carvacrol and thymol are "a perfect example of the advantages natural substances hold over synthetic ones."[43]

To ensure the safe use of oregano oil with cats, AVOID the following:

- Undiluted essential oils, either internally or topically (look for brands that are diluted specifically for pet use);

- Chemically-extracted essential oils (look for brands that are all-natural and steam-distilled, without the use of chemical solvents);

- Non-dietary oils, like cedar oil and tea tree oil, either internally or topically;

- Large doses of any essential oil (cats are smaller and more sensitive to essential oils);

- Daily use of any essential oil (including oregano oil) without a break (10 days on and two days off may be suitable);

- Any essential oil if you are not 100 percent sure about its safety. If in doubt, don't use it.

5

Success with Oil of Oregano

Of all the information I can present supporting the use of Oil of Oregano, perhaps the most convincing evidence comes directly from the thousands of people who have benefited from its practical uses in their daily lives.

The stories below are first-hand accounts from people describing, in their own words, how they have used Oil of Oregano for a wide assortment of health issues. Reading these should give you a better idea of just how amazing Oil of Oregano truly is. Many thanks to *Joy of the Mountains*, who shared their product testimonials with us.

COLDS AND FLUS

Cold and Flu Prevention

Since I discovered Oil of Oregano, I am not getting sick anymore. I run a daycare at home so I am always in contact with germs, viruses, etc. As soon as I feel that I might be coming down with a cold or the flu, I take my Oil of Oregano and 'boom', it is gone!!! *Mélissa L., Gatineau, QC*

Cold and Flu Symptoms

When I begin to feel the onset of cold or flu-like symptoms, I take Joy of the Mountains Oil of Oregano - it stops my cold from developing every time. I tell everybody about the benefits of Oil of Oregano, and I always recommend Joy of the Mountains! *Lisa C., Victoria, BC*

Cold, Flu, Earache, and Inflammation

I had the flu/cold recently, and developed an earache, with such pain and inflammation I could barely speak or eat which normally would have sent me to the Doctor for an antibiotic. Luckily I had Oil of Oregano at home, so I began to take this. Within two days I noticed my earache pain vanished and so did the inflammation! I trust this product and recommend to all. *Samantha W., R.M.T. Calgary, AB*

Cold, Flu, Sinus Issues, and Allergies

I swear by Joy of the Mountains. I promote it in the workplace for anyone with a cold, flu, sinus issues or allergies. After using antibiotics for three months for a sinus infection, I was introduced to your product by a health food store. It cleared up within three days. I use it now as a preventative (when my grandchildren are visiting and sick with colds). As soon as I feel a cold coming on, I take it promptly and have avoided a full-blown cold and/or sinus infection. *Christine B., Sherbrooke, QC*

Cold, Flu, Immune Support, and Candida

As a Clinical Herbalist, I've had a lot of opportunity to see what works best when it comes to fighting infections, naturally. Top of the list? Oil of Oregano. Whether it's for preventative immune support, or for dealing with an acute infection such as cold or flu after it has arisen, Oil of Oregano works quickly and reliably. It's also indispensable for helping to address intestinal Candida (yeast) overgrowth and chronic infectious conditions. Oregano oil's broad-spectrum action makes it uniquely effective against a wide variety of organisms—bacteria, viruses, fungi and yeast, and parasites. With the increasingly virulent and drug-resistant germs developing nowadays, Oil of Oregano is more important than ever. I recommend that everyone have it on hand. *Paulina N., RH (AHG), Vancouver, BC*

Cough and Cold

All winter I've managed to survive without getting sick, but recently with the unbearable ever-changing weather here in Toronto, I finally got a cold. I've been skeptical about buying this product, but said what the heck, $20, will give it a try. After following the directions I took the Oil of Oregano and it's almost like a miracle, I can't believe how much better I feel with the cough nearly non-existent. Thank you so much for a great product. The fact that it's Canadian makes it even better. Thank you, Joy of the Mountains! *Martin N, Mississauga, ON*

General Health and Immune Booster

We have been taking Oil of Oregano daily for several months now, and our doctor has given us a clean bill of health. We had blood work done and according to the doc we don't have high cholesterol, our immune systems are very strong... I personally believe it's because of the oil. Both Geoff and I have had great results from using it. Colds only last for a few days if we even get them at all! Also, my skin has cleared up since I've started using the product. I highly recommend it as a daily preventative. We enjoy the taste of it and actually crave it. Thank you for such a top quality product. *Kari and Geoff N., Lethbridge, AB*

RESPIRATORY AND SINUS CONDITIONS

Bronchitis and Chronic Cough

I have had recurring bronchitis for years, and a chronic annoying cough that never seems to go away. Prescriptions proved ineffective, including two different types of inhalers. When I heard about the effects of Oil of Oregano on bronchitis, I immediately tried Joy of the Mountains. Within two weeks, my bronchitis completely disappeared! Now I take the oil as I need to. Sometimes that annoying cough returns, and when it does, your Oil of Oregano works every time! *Jay O., Victoria, BC*

Continuous Sneezing/Draining Sinuses

Recently, I felt a cold coming on strong with continuous sneezing and draining sinuses... I took Oil of Oregano internally (orally), but I also mixed five drops with a cup of boiling water. I placed my head over the cup with a towel covering me and inhaled the fumes through my nose and mouth, just like my mother used to have me do with menthol when I was a child. I did this for about 10 minutes. I went to bed right after this treatment and when I woke up the next morning all symptoms were gone and I felt fine. It was the shortest cold I have ever experienced, less than 24 hours. I have experienced so many benefits from Oil of Oregano that I cannot help sharing this with my friends and co-workers when they tell me of a problem. Needless to say, I have won over many of them who were skeptical until they tried it. *Ian M., Orleans, ON*

Pneumonia

I've been using Oil of Oregano for four years and have had great results every time with the product. A year ago, my mother had pneumonia for three weeks. I told her about Oil of Oregano and she decided to use it, and to her surprise she was almost all clear within 12 hours. In three days all symptoms of her pneumonia were gone. She is now a very firm believer in Oil of Oregano. And since that time, I have brought many of my co-workers on board. Thank you, Joy of the Mountains!
Frank D., Hinton, AB

Pneumonia, Cough, and Airborne Viruses

I picked up a bottle of Joy of the Mountains Oil of Oregano last Tuesday. I have had pneumonia from Christmas to mid-January and a cough ever since. I've tried antibiotics, Cold-FX, inhalers, etc. Finally this past Friday I decided to try your product. IT WORKED! Although my sinuses are still a little stuffed up, I have been cough-free now since Saturday, for the first time this year. I have been so thrilled with the results. Oil of Oregano has become a staple in my medicine cabinet at home. As a matter of fact, I carry a small bottle in my purse and make use of it when travelling, as airplanes can be full of airborne viruses. Thank you and keep up the good work.
Anne B., Gatineau, QC

Sinus Infection

It was suggested to me to try Oil of Oregano for an oncoming sinus infection. I was on it two days and it was gone. I was thrilled, so I continued to take it as a preventative measure.
Coralee B., St. Albert, AB

Sinus Issues

My husband has a bad sinus problem and was constantly taking Dristan, or similar products. I couldn't wear perfume around him or he'd immediately stuff right up and couldn't breathe properly. Going from cold outside to a warm restaurant, he stuffed right up and couldn't taste his meal. Upon learning about Oil of Oregano, he decided to give it a try. He took two drops a day, and with three weeks the change was incredible. I can now wear perfume, and he can breathe! *Vicki N., Kamloops, BC*

SKIN CONDITIONS

Chronic Nail Fungus

Toenail fungus has stubbornly plagued me for over 20 years, and absolutely nothing has worked against it. I finally heard about the natural antibiotic effect of Oil of Oregano and started applying drops directly under the toenails. I was amazed. Within two months I was actually seeing improvement, after years of trying all other options to no avail. All I can say is that I'm no longer embarrassed to wear sandals in public and my nails are looking pink and healthy again. Thank you, Joy of the Mountains! *Carol C., Penticton, BC*

Chronic Skin Condition

For the past six months I have been using your Oil of Oregano. It was recommended to me at a gathering of 60+ folks. I have a skin condition that is 40 years old. I have been to countless medical and naturopathic practitioners. None have been able to diagnose it to date. I have taken all sorts of natural and chemical prescribed medications. The only product that has provided me with any relief to date has been Joy of the Mountains Oil of Oregano. No, it has not cured my condition, but it has been effective in clearing up my skin. Just so you know the extent of my condition, it virtually covers all of my body with the exception of my face. I am confident that with continued use, it will gradually improve a 40-year fight to better looking skin. I have shared my experience with many people so they too may experience better overall health. Keep up your good work. *Roy K., Vernon, BC*

Head Lice/Nits

My daughter got head lice at school and lucky me, I caught it from her. I visited your website for treatment information. I used a full bottle of Oil of Oregano and mixed it with olive oil 1:1. I diligently put the mixture on our scalps for five days, removing any lice or nits I found. (We still have the mixture in case of a next time.) The "burning" sensation was non-existent for me. For my daughter who has sensitive skin, she did notice the "burn" at a 1:1 dilution but it wasn't uncomfortable. I have used the oil undiluted on my own skin with no problem, but if I use it undiluted on my daughter, her skin turns red and itchy. This was part of the reason I followed the instructions and diluted 1:1. I did not notice the scalp turning red on either of us, though my daughter did have some reddish color at the base of her neck. We both slept with the product in, we put a towel on our pillow. No product got into our eyes. I did not find any more live lice after two days and no nits after three days; however I wanted to 'make sure and continued for five days. We are now free (of head lice) and have wonderful conditioned hair as a bonus. Plus we always smelled like pizza, which is a good thing. We use your product for so much and I was happy to find out, once more, that Mother Nature provided a remedy instead of having to use a pesticide. I have already spoken with the principal of my daughter's school and the health nurse who does the regular lice checks at the school. They are restricted to "tried and true" shampoos, etc. as far as the printed paperwork that goes out once lice has been detected in a classroom. However, woman-to-woman, I am sure the word will spread that Oil of Oregano is an alternative method that has worked for us. *Edina K., Kelowna, BC*

Nail Fungus and Pet Care

Just wanted to let you know that you have a great product. My husband has used it to treat fungus in his big toes and now we are treating a bladder infection in our miniature schnauzer. *Bernice, Vancouver, BC*

Nail Fungus, Toothache, and Chapped Lips

We came from Germany and we found "Oil of Oregano" and we would like to say - thank you - it is a very good oil for whatever. We used it for nail fungus (Nagelpilz-Infektion) and Toothache ... With the nail fungus I went in Germany to a doctor, but nothing helps me! Now, with Oil of Oregano, the fungus is gone. I was able to help and introduce more friends with Oil of Oregano. One of them is a welder and works outside on farms and his lips were very dry and painful. Only one drop of Oil of Oregano in a little bit of Melkfett or other cream and it helps right away. He is so happy and will buy his own bottle now. Last week I went with students from my English class to the local health food store, and they bought Oil of Oregano after I told them how good this is! *Karl T., AB*

Toenail Fungus

I had toenail fungus on both feet and after using a daily drop of Joy of the Mountains Oil of Oregano on them for a few months, they are totally clear and I have not had any further problems. My mother, who had been in Assisted Living, had not had good foot care. She had toenail fungus so bad that the nails were curled. They are clearing up with the same treatment. *Sandra F., Hendersonville, NC*

SORE MUSCLES AND JOINTS

Fibromyalgia

Hello, my name is Nabu. I am a six year Fibromyalgia sufferer. My hands are so stiff in the morning I have to soak them in hot water with Oil of Oregano just to use them. Over the years I have tried everything, and I mean everything: Diet, herbs, even morphine. The pain in my body is bigger than all of these. Without the morphine I just can't get out of bed at all. Cold weather is very hard on me. Yet, with your Oil of Oregano massaged onto my legs, arms and neck, I can take less morphine and do not fear the morning pain. Imagine, hurting all over constantly. Your Oil of Oregano has been turning my life around. Thank you so much for this improvement. My unbelievable suffering has seemed to lift... I have obtained results that pulled me out of my wheelchair and allow me to walk with a walker. Thank you so very much! *Nabu B., Bellingham, WA*

Sore Joints and Injured Muscles

Not only is Oil of Oregano effective against infections - it is an anti-inflammatory and helps to reduce pain when applied topically. I recommend it for sore joints and injured muscles, and to speed the healing of any type of wound. *Julie M., R.M.T. Summerland, BC*

Sore Muscles and Cough/Cold

Wow, am I so glad I found out about Joy of the Mountains Oil of Oregano. I use it on my daughter for her sore muscles; I massage it into the affected area and it relieves her pain. I also used it for my own nagging cough due to cold. I can also sleep at night when I take my Oil of Oregano. Thanks! *Cathy W., Port Coquitlam, BC*

Sprained Ankle

When I sprained my ankle I got out my Oil of Oregano and put it on. It was very helpful because the next day I was able to walk okay ... it was bruised but I was able to get around on my own two feet. Thanks to Oil of Oregano!! *Val O., Red Deer, AB*

BURNS, WOUNDS, CUTS, BRUISES, AND BLISTERS

Burn Injury

This is amazing stuff. I spilled a cup of hot boiling tea water all over my left hand at work two days ago. The top of my thumb received most of the damage, the skin was red and irritated and hot and it hurt a lot. I was afraid that it would start to blister so I kept running cold water over it. It felt okay, but as soon as I stopped doing that it would hurt a lot. I walked down to my health food store with a wet paper towel over my thumb. The owner of the shop asked what was wrong. She immediately told me about Joy of the Mountains Oil of Oregano. She took the sampler and put one single tiny drop on my burned skin. I let it soak in for a few minutes and gently rubbed it into the skin. Amazingly, within 15-20 minutes I didn't feel any pain at all. Just one single application did the trick. The skin did not blister, did not scar, and did not peel off. Next morning I was having a hot shower like nothing happened. Unbelievable product. *Jay G., Calgary, AB*

Cut/Wound

My cut did not heal even after seven days, I put Polysporin and nothing. After that I decided to put one drop of oregano oil and in the morning I could not believe my wound was closed and healing. From that time I always carry my oregano and use it for everything. *Madja, Vancouver, BC*

Cuts, Sore Joints, and Colds

I've used Oil of Oregano on cuts that were serious and the healing process is amazing. Our family uses Oil of Oregano for all sorts of things from sore joints to colds. Works great and is a great natural alternative. We've used Joy of the Mountains for over two years now. *Marcus H., Calgary, AB*

Oil Burn

I just burnt myself on the arm with very hot oil. I immediately put Oil of Oregano on the burn to reduce the pain and inflammation. No water blister formed, and one week later my skin is already regenerating!!! *Mélissa L., Gatineau, QC*

MOUTH CONDITIONS

Dental Hygiene

I put Joy of the Mountains Oil of Oregano on my toothbrush once a day. My teeth feel like I just had them cleaned at the dentist! My dental hygienist said, "Whatever you are doing, keep doing it." *Debra S., Burns Lake, BC*

Tooth and Gum Health

I use Joy of the Mountains as an everyday mouthwash. Because it does the best job of killing bacteria, it's great for keeping my gums healthy and my breath fresh. I have a tooth that has been "iffy" since root canal surgery. Whenever it starts aching, I know some bacteria have gotten up inside. All I have to do is spread Joy of the Mountains around the tooth, take a few doses internally, and the infection goes away. It has saved my tooth. *Susan P., Vancouver, BC*

DIGESTIVE CONDITIONS

Celiac Disease, IBS, and Leg Pain

I suffer from Celiac disease, IBS and leg pain, but since using Joy of the Mountains my symptoms have greatly diminished. The leg pain has gone completely. *Roz C., Vernon, BC*

Colitis

Just wanted to drop a quick note to say wild oregano is a wonderful product to use for everything. I discovered it after reading Jini Patel Thompson's book Listen to your Gut as I have colitis. When I am having a flare-up, out comes the oil as well as other natural products. It does take a while to "take hold" as per all natural products, but it does make my symptoms improve heaps. *Debbie, Sydney, Australia*

IBD, Sinus Issues, and Aching Joints

I started taking your Oil of Oregano for my Inflammatory Bowel Disease. In about two weeks I noticed a big difference. Then I noticed I could breathe through both nostrils... something I haven't been able to do for years. I also noticed my aching joints had improved a lot. I take five to 10 drops in a small amount of olive oil two to three times a day... Thank you for this wonderful product. It is now a part of my life. *Carl C., Abbotsford, BC*

IBS and Stomach Discomfort/Gas

As a result of taking it regularly, the Irritable Bowel Syndrome (IBS) I have had at least 10 years is completely GONE. I can eat foods I haven't for years; I am not plagued by stomach discomfort or gas. I feel normal again!!!!! *Coralee B., St. Albert, AB*

Upset Stomach

I have been using Joy of the Mountains Oil of Oregano for about six months ever since a natural pharmacist recommended it for an upset stomach. I have found it to be as effective as the claims I have read. *Ian M., Orleans, ON*

INFECTION-RELATED CONDITIONS

Leg Infection

I have been taking Oil of Oregano for over a year now, since my last leg operation. Before then I kept getting an infection in the left leg, which I could not get rid of, the infection kept coming back. A year later and the leg has never felt so good. I do not need to put the oil on the knee anymore, as the last CAT scan confirmed that there was no infection in the bone, and everything is healed up. Thank you for the Oil of Oregano product, I would say it saved my life. I was on other drugs in the hospital, but the Oil of Oregano did the trick. A very happy person! *Arthur F., Mount Hope, ON*

Otitis

My son has recurring otitis, and woke up one morning with a fever and an earache. I rubbed Oil of Oregano behind his ear, and the next morning it was gone. Thank you for this oil; I don't know what I would do without it!!! *Mélissa L., Gatineau, QC*

Shingles

I was introduced to Joy of the Mountains Oil of Oregano while I had shingles. I was advised by my family physician that the pain could last for up to 10 years! No word of a lie, the very next day after my first topical treatment of Oil of Oregano, I could feel the pain lessen. Within two or three days the pain was completely gone—that was three and a half years ago. Made a believer out of me! *Patti S., High Level, AB*

Toe Infection

I ripped a cuticle on my toe and it caused a serious infection; my foot was swollen, red and warm and I could not sleep anymore. I then thought about the oil. I put a drop on it, and what a miracle—I woke up the next morning and it was all gone. *Mélissa L., Gatineau, QC*

Wart Removal

Can Oil of Oregano remove warts? It did for me. Wash the area, apply a drop of Oil of Oregano directly on the wart, and cover with a bandage to keep the oil in contact with the wart. Leave the bandage on as long as possible. When the bandage comes off, repeat the previous steps. Continue until the wart is gone. There is no discomfort of any kind. Oil of Oregano is a natural cure. *Leigh M., New Westminster, BC*

Warts on Hands/Feet

I am so thrilled! My young daughter injured her foot over a year ago, and warts developed at the injury site. These spread onto her hands and her other foot within only a few months! We tried all the bottled wart removers to no avail. Then we heard about Oil of Oregano, and I read that it can help warts. She started right away, applying the oil at night, and wearing mittens and socks to bed, and in two months, the warts are all gone!!! I mean it, they are all gone! Thank you, Joy of the Mountains! My daughter is no longer ashamed to show her hands and feet! *Mary Jane C.*

IMPROVED SLEEP

Sleep Issues

Our seniors in the community are intrigued with healthy cures they can have on hand. One lady, who owns a local deli, hasn't slept for more than two hours at a time, for a long time. She started using your Oil of Oregano and immediately started sleeping for at least four hours. *Judy R., ON*

PET CARE

Sores and Skin Problems

My almost 13-year-old Shih Tzu/Poodle has developed some skin problems, which is common to that breed at this age. One sore was wide open exposing her flesh. I applied the OregaPet First Aid Gel one time and noticed a great improvement in the healing of the sore. The second application totally closed over the sore and it has cleared right up. This surprised me... it worked extremely well and I am happy to have a natural product that works — and saves me a ton of money in vet bills! *Rene G., BC*

Pet Odors and Skin Issues

I love the OregaPet Bed & Body Spray. For one thing it smells wonderful and I would use it in my bathroom and kitchen in a heartbeat. A friend dropped in one day when I had used it and she said, "What is that great smell?" Of course I told her it was OregaPet. I have used it to freshen up my doggy smelling car with great results. I have used it on her body when her skin seemed dry and I spray it on her just because I love the smell. Have also used it in her bed when she has had skin issues and I have to say that her skin problems are almost cleared up... *Catherine M., BC*

Flea Treatment for Cats

My wife and I live in Vilcabamba, Ecuador, and have three cats. Vilcabamba, for those who don't know, is a haven of beauty and natural splendour... and that is why we moved here. Accordingly, we hardly use chemicals for anything at all, and certainly did not want to poison our cats with conventional flea treatments. So when we discovered OregaPet, it was a godsend! We have been treating our cats with OregaPet Bed & Body Spray for two months now, and their fleas have disappeared. Our cats are now even happier than they were before! And that makes us happy. We recommend all pet owners try OregaPet for themselves. Why use chemicals if you can harness the natural benefits of oregano oil products? *Nick V. and Laura A., Vilcabamba, Ecuador*

Flea Treatment for Dog

Hey, the flea stuff OregaPet Bed & Body Spray is a huge hit! I gave it to one of the kids at the shelter for his Pit Bull puppy, and he said it worked in 20 minutes, killed them all and they never came back — yay! So tell whoever makes it that it's great! *Natalie S., Victoria, BC*

Swollen Gums/Bad Breath

I have been giving my Shih Tzu/Poodle, Annie, a few drops of oil of oregano on a piece of rice cake with a bit of butter and almond butter. She is a bit cautious as the oil is strong but she actually licks it all off the cracker. I wonder if she knows that her body needs this? She had swollen gums and very bad breath and after a couple of doses her breath improved by 50 percent. That has been so encouraging to me. She probably has some inflammatory problems and I know from my own experience, being a senior as well, that oil of oregano helps the whole body. I am so thankful for OregaPet — we are the "oregano girls!" *Rene G., BC*

Lice Prevention

I picked up two bottles of OregaPet Bed & Body Spray from you a few weeks ago. I brought my two Min Pins (Mickey and Minnie) to daycare twice and sprayed them. They got lots of sniffing attention from the other dogs. I also sprayed them when we got together with a neighbor's dog who had had a problem with lice. Mickey and Minnie have been clear every time. I will continue to use the product when I feel they could be exposed. If you don't hear from me, all is well. *Marie, Kelowna, BC*

Skin Problems/Allergies

There are so many skin problems/allergies with Bulldogs! Our's (Mia) is seven months old, and she recently started to limp. We thought she hurt her paw, and then we figured out she had cracked paws. We do not know the cause (it could be the weather in the winter, salt/sand combo, heat, allergies, or chemicals). We are now using a green floor cleaner to eliminate the chemicals. We also needed to find something safe as she will lick her paws. We started using OregaPet First Aid Gel twice a day for eight days and her paws healed up and she stopped limping! I'm going to tell my Vet about OregaPet. Thank you, this is a great "safe" product! *Stacy M., BC*

Considerations

When using Oil of Oregano to overcome infections or other conditions, there are a few important points to be considered.

Always ensure that your oregano oil products come from a trusted source and are made with genuine, unadulterated essential oil. The oil should be certified organic or wild-harvested to ensure there are no pesticides or chemicals. Make sure the carvacrol is naturally-occurring, along with the plant's other beneficial phytochemicals. Also be certain that you are using a safely diluted Oil of Oregano product and not pure, undiluted oregano essential oil.

Another thing to consider is the use of complementary supplements. Enzymes and probiotics are very beneficial to use together with Oil of Oregano. Enzymes assist in the absorption of many of the active phytochemical properties of oregano, helping to increase their effectiveness when Oil of Oregano is taken orally. Probiotics will help increase the levels of your "friendly bacteria," which can become decreased due to infection or antibiotic drugs. As a general safeguard, take a good quality probiotic for a few weeks after any antibiotic use, to help restore balance in your intestinal tract.

I hope this guide has inspired hope for those who may be suffering from a chronic illness, and for which oregano oil may be of benefit. Please share the knowledge you have gained so that enlightenment may encourage change within our current healthcare system, and common sense may rule our judgment once again.

References

In-Text Citations

1 World Health Organization (WHO), 2013a

2 European Centre for Disease Prevention and Control (ECDC), 2012a

3 ECDC, 2012b

4 Infectious Diseases Society of America (IDSA), 2004; Levine, 2006, pp. S5-S12; Klevens et al., 2007b, pp.1763-1771

5 Klevens et al., 2007a, pp.160-166

6 Guggenbichler, Assadian, Boeswald, & Kramer, 2011, Doc18

7 WHO, 2012

8 IDSA, 2004; Interagency Task Force on Antimicrobial Resistance (ITFAR), 2012

9 Centers for Disease Control and Prevention (CDC), 2002-2009

10 WHO, 2009c; WHO, 2013b

11 WHO, 2009c

12 WHO, 2012

13 IDSA, 2004

14 WHO, 2011

15 Coates, Halls & Hu, 2011, pp. 184-194; IDSA, 2004

16 WHO, 2012

17 Buhner, 1999; Kades, 2005

[18] Nikaido, 2009, pp. 119-146; Wise, 2002, pp. 585–586

[19] Lappé, 1986

[20] Al-Bahry et al., 2009, pp. 720-725

[21] Perencevich, Wong, & Harris, 2001, pp. 281-283

[22] Lapen et al., 2008, pp. 50-65; Fair et al., 2009, pp. 2248-2254; Baier-Anderon & Monosson, 2008; John Hopkins Bloomberg School of Public Health, 2005

[23] CDC, 2013

[24] Harth, 2010; Calafat, Ye, Wong, Reidy, & Needham, 2008, pp. 303–307

[25] Natural Resources Defense Council, 2011; Natural Resources Defense Council, 2010

[26] Brehm, 2011

[27] Subbiah, Shah, Besser, Ullman, & Call, 2012, e48919

[28] Joint Expert Technical Advisory Committee on Antibiotic Resistance (JETACAR), 1999

[29] Smillie, et al., 2011, December, pp. 241–244; O'Brien, 2002, pp. S78-S84; Norberg, Bergström, Jethava, Dubhashi, and Hermansson, 2011, p. 68

[30] Resistance Genes in Our Food Supply, 2007

[31] Zhang, Zhang, & Fang, 2009, pp. 397-414; Xi et al., 2009, pp. 5714–5718; Forsberg, et al., 2012, pp. 1107-1111; Yang et al., 2013

[32] Buhner, 1999

[33] JETACAR, 1999

[34] Georgetown University Medical Center, 2001

[35] Elgayyar, Draughon, Golden, & Mount, 2001, pp. 1019-1024

[36] University of the West of England, 2008

[37] Hammer, Carson, & Riley, 1999, pp. 985–990

[38] Dorman, H. J. D., & Deans, S.G. (2000, February). Antimicrobial agents from plants: Antibacterial activity of plant volatile oils. Journal of Applied Microbiology, 88 (2), 308-316.

[39] Schnaubelt, 1998

[40] Schnaubelt, 1998

[41] Vimalanathan, S., & Hudson, J. (2012)

[42] University of the West of England, 2008

[43] Schnaubelt, 1998

Full References

Alanis, A.J. (2005). Resistance to antibiotics: Are we in the post-antibiotic era? *Archives of Medical Research*, 36(6), 697-705. doi:10.1016/j.arcmed.2005.06.009

Al-Bahry, S., Mahmoud, I., Elshafie, A., Al-Harthy, A., Al-Ghafri, S., Al-Amri, I., & Alkindi, A. (2009, May). Bacterial flora and antibiotic resistance from eggs of green turtles Chelonia mydas: An indication of polluted effluents. *Marine Pollution Bulletin*, 58(5), 720-725. doi:10.1016/j.marpolbul.2008.12.018

Aristatile, B., Al-Numair, K.S., Al-Assaf, A.H., & Pugalendi, K.V. (2011). Pharmacological effect of carvacrol on D: -galactosamine-induced mitochondrial enzymes and DNA damage by single-cell gel electrophoresis. *Journal of Natural Medicines*, 65(3-4), 568-577.

Atanda, O.O., Akpan I., & Oluwafemi F. (2007). The potential of some spice essential oils in the control of A. parasiticus CFR 223 and aflatoxin production. *Food Control*, 18(5), 601-607. doi:10.1016/j.foodcont.2006.02.007

Australian Broadcasting Corporation (ABC). (1999). *What Can We Do?* Retrieved from http://www.abc.net.au/science/slab/antibiotics/what_to_do.htm

Aydin, S., & Seker, E. (2005). Effect of an aqueous distillate of Origanum onites L. on isolated rat fundus, duodenum and ileum: Evidence for the role of oxygenated monoterpenes. *Pharmazie*, 60(2), 147-50.

Baier-Anderon, C., & Monosson, E. (2008, December 5). Triclosan and triclocarban in consumer products. *The Encyclopedia of Earth*. Retrieved from http://www.eoearth.org/

Bendini, A., Toschi T.G., & Lercker G. (2002). Antioxidant activity of oregano (Origanum vulgare L.) leaves. *Italian Journal of Food Science, 14*, 17–23.

Braga, P.C., Dal Sasso, M., Culici, M., Bianchi, T., Bordoni, L., & Marabini, L. (2006). Anti-inflammatory activity of thymol: Inhibitory effect on the release of human neutrophil elastase. *Pharmacology, 77*, 130-136. doi:10.1159/000093790

Brehm, D. (2011, October 30). Bacteria may readily swap beneficial genes. *MIT News*. Retrieved from http://web.mit.edu/newsoffice/

Buhner, S.H. (1999). *Herbal antibiotics: Natural alternatives for treating drug-resistant bacteria.* Pownal, VT: Storey Books.

Burt, S. (2004). Essential oils: Their antibacterial properties and potential applications in foods–a review. *International Journal of Food Microbiology, 94*, 223-253. doi:10.1016/j.ijfoodmicro.2004.03.022

Burt, S.A., & Reinders, R.D. (2003). Antibacterial activity of selected plant essential oils against Escherichia coli O157:H7. *Letters in Applied Microbiology, 36*(3), 162-167. doi:10.1111/j.1365-2672.2005.02789.x

Calafat, A.M., Ye, X., Wong, L., Reidy, J.A., & Needham, L.L. (2008, March). Urinary concentrations of triclosan in the U.S. population: 2003–2004. *Environmental Health Perspectives, 116*(3), 303–307. doi:10.1289/ehp.10768

Centers for Disease Control and Prevention. (1995). *Recommendations for preventing the spread of vancomycin resistance: Recommendations of the Hospital Infection Control Practices Advisory Committee (HICPAC).* Retrieved from http://www.cdc.gov/

Centers for Disease Control and Prevention. (2002-2009). *West Nile virus: Statistics, surveillance, and control archive.* Retrieved from http://www.cdc.gov/

Centers for Disease Control and Prevention. (2010a). *The 2009 H1N1 pandemic: Summary highlights, April 2009-April 2010.* Retrieved from http://www.cdc.gov/

Centers for Disease Control and Prevention. (2010b). *Updated CDC estimates of 2009 H1N1 influenza cases, hospitalizations and deaths in the United States, April 2009-April 2010.* Retrieved from http://www.cdc.gov/

Centers for Disease Control and Prevention. (2011). *Diseases and organisms in healthcare settings.* Retrieved from http://www.cdc.gov/

Centers for Disease Control and Prevention. (2012). *Influenza antiviral drug resistance.* Retrieved from http://www.cdc.gov/

Centers for Disease Control and Prevention. (2013a). *Carbapenem-resistant enterobacteriaceae (CRE).* Retrieved from http://www.cdc.gov/

Centers for Disease Control and Prevention. (2013b). *National report on human exposure to environmental chemicals.* Retrieved from http://www.cdc.gov/

Chami, N., Chami, F., Bennis, S., Trouillas, J., & Remmal, A. (2004). Antifungal treatment with carvacrol and eugenol of oral candidiasis in immunosuppressed rats. *Brazilian Journal of Infectious Diseases, 8*(3), 217-226.

Coates, A.R., Halls, G., & Hu Y. (2011, May). Novel classes of antibiotics or more of the same? *British Journal of Pharmacology, 163*(1), 184-194. doi:10.1111/j.1476-5381.2011.01250.x

Conly, J., & Johnston, B. (2005, May). Where are all the new antibiotics? The new antibiotic paradox. *The Canadian Journal of Infectious Diseases & Medical Microbiology, 16*(3), 159–160.

Dorman, H. J. D., & Deans, S.G. (2000, February). Antimicrobial agents from plants: Antibacterial activity of plant volatile oils. *Journal of Applied Microbiology, 88*(2), 308-316.

Duke, J.A. (1997). *The green pharmacy: New discoveries in herbal remedies for common diseases and conditions from the world's foremost authority on healing herbs.* Emmaus, PA: Rodale Press.

Eber, M.R., Laxminarayan, R., Perencevich, E.N., & Malani, A. (2010). Clinical and economic outcomes attributable to health care-associated sepsis and pneumonia. *Archives of Internal Medicine, 170*(4), 347-353. doi:10.1001/archinternmed.2009.509

Elgayyar, M., Draughon, F.A., Golden, D.A., & Mount, J.R. (2001, July). Antimicrobial activity of essential oils from plants against selected pathogenic and saprophytic microorganisms. *Journal of Food Protection, 64*(7), 1019-1024.

European Centre for Disease Prevention and Control. (2012a). *Antimicrobial resistance surveillance in Europe 2011. Annual report of the European Antimicrobial Resistance Surveillance Network (EARS-Net).* Stockholm: ECDC. doi:10.2900/14911

European Centre for Disease Prevention and Control. (2012b, November 16). *Multidrug antibiotic resistance increasing in Europe.* Retrieved from http://ecdc.europa.eu/

Fair, P.A., Lee, H., Adams, J., Darling, C., Pacepavicius, G., Alaee, M., . . . Muir, D. (2009). Occurrence of triclosan in plasma of wild Atlantic bottlenose dolphins (Tursiops truncatus) and in their environment. *Environmental Pollution, 157*(8-9), 2248-2254. doi:10.1016/j.envpol.2009.04.002

Fontaine, D. (2010, May). *Shopping for health: A buyer's guide to oil of oregano* [Corporate brochure].

Force, M., Sparks, W.S., & Ronzio, R.A. (2000). Inhibition of enteric parasites by emulsified oil of oregano in vivo. *Phytotherapy Research, 14*(3), 213-214.

Forsberg, K.J., Reyes, A., Wang, B., Selleck, E.M., Sommer, M.O.A., & Dantas, G. (2012, August 31). The shared antibiotic resistome of soil bacteria and human pathogens. *Science, 337*(6098), 1107-1111. doi:10.1126/science.1220761

Georgetown University Medical Center. (2001, October 11). Oregano oil may protect against drug-resistant bacteria, Georgetown researcher finds. *Science Daily.* Retrieved from http://www.sciencedaily.com/

Grolle, J., & Hackenbroch, V. (2009, July 21). Interview with epidemiologist Tom Jefferson: A whole industry is waiting for a pandemic. *Der Spiegel.* Retrieved from http://www.spiegel.de/

Guggenbichler, J.P., Assadian, O., Boeswald, M., & Kramer, A. (2011). Incidence and clinical implication of nosocomial infections associated with implantable biomaterials—catheters, ventilator-associated pneumonia, urinary tract infections. GMS *Krankenhhyg Interdiszip, 6*(1), Doc18. doi:10.3205/dgkh000175

Hammer, K.A., Carson, C.F., & Riley, T.V. (1999, June). Antimicrobial activity of essential oils and other plant extracts. *Journal of Applied Microbiology, 86*(6), 985–990.

Harth, R. (2010, November 9). *Myth of a germ-free world: A closer look at antimicrobial products.* Tempe, AZ: Biodesign Institute at ASU. Retrieved from http://www.biodesign.asu.edu/

Ijaz, M.K., Chen, Z., Raja, S.S., Suchmann, D.B., Royt, P.W., Ingram, C., . . . Paolilli, G. (2004). Antiviral and virucidal activities of oreganol P73-based spice extracts against human coronavirus in vitro. International Conference on Antiviral Research (XVII), *Antiviral Research, Abstracts, 62*(2), 121.

Infectious Diseases Society of America (IDSA). (2004). *Bad bugs, no drugs: As antibiotic discovery stagnates... a public health crisis brews.* Retrieved from http://www.fda.gov/

Infectious Diseases Society of America (IDSA). (2010, June). *Antibiotic resistance: Promoting critically needed antibiotic research and development and appropriate use ("stewardship") of these precious drugs.* Retrieved from http://www.idsociety.org/

Ingram, C. (2001). *Wild oregano oil: Ancient remedy, modern research.* Retrieved from http://www.kombuchahealth.com.au

Ingram, C. (2008). *The cure is in the cupboard: How to use oregano for better health.* Buffalo Grove, IL: Knowledge House Publishers.

Interagency Task Force on Antimicrobial Resistance (ITFAR). (2012). *A public health action plan to combat antimicrobial resistance: 2012 update.* Retrieved from http://www.cdc.gov/

Jayakumar, S., Madankumar, A., Asokkumar, S., Raghunandhakumar, S., Gokula Dhas, K., Kamaraj, S., . . . Devaki, T. (2012). Potential preventive effect of carvacrol against diethylnitrosamine-induced hepatocellular carcinoma in rats. *Molecular and Cellular Biochemistry, 360*(1-2), 51-60. doi:10.1007/s11010-011-1043-7

John Hopkins Bloomberg School of Public Health. (2005, December 23). *Cleaning up antimicrobial hand soaps* [Interview with Dr. Rolf Halden]. Retrieved from http://www.jhsph.edu/

Joint Expert Technical Advisory Committee on Antibiotic Resistance (JETACAR). (1999, October). *The use of antibiotics in food producing animals: Antibiotic-resistant bacteria in animals and humans.* Retrieved from http://www.health.gov.au/

Kades, E. (2005). Preserving a precious resource: Rationalizing the use of antibiotics. *Faculty Publications, Paper 52.* Retrieved from http://scholarship.law.wm.edu/

Klevens, R.M., Edwards, J.R., Richards, C.L., Jr., Horan, T.C., Gaynes, R.P., Pollock, D.A., & Cardo, D.M. (2007a). Estimating health care-associated infections and deaths in U.S. hospitals, 2002. *Public Health Reports, 122*(2), 160-166.

Klevens, R.M., Morrison, M.A., Nadle, J., Petit, S., Gershman, K., Ray, S., . . . Fridkin, S.K. (2007b, October 17). Invasive methicillin-resistant staphylococcus aureus infections in the United States. *Journal of the American Medical Association, 298*(15), 1763-1771.

Lagatolla, C., Tonin, E.A., Monti-Bragadin, C., Dolzani, L., Gombac, F., Bearzi, C., . . . Rossolini, G.M. (2004). Endemic carbapenem-resistant Pseudomonas aeruginosa with acquired metallo-B-lactamase determinants in European hospital. *Emerging Infectious Diseases, 10*(3), 535-538. doi:10.1001/jama.298.15.1763

Lambert, R.J., Skandamis, P.N., Coote, P.J., & Nychas, G.J. (2001). A study of the minimum inhibitory concentration and mode of action of oregano essential oil, thymol and carvacrol. *Journal of Applied Microbiology, 91*(3), 453-462.

Lapen, D.R., Topp, E., Metcalfe, C.D., Li, H., Edwards, M., Gottschall, N., . . . Beck, A. (2008). Pharmaceutical and personal care products in tile drainage following land application of municipal biosolids. *The Science of the Total Environment, 399*(1-3), 50-65. doi:10.1016/j.scitotenv.2008.02.025

Lappé, M. (1986). *When antibiotics fail: Restoring the ecology of the body.* Berkeley, CA: North Atlantic Books.

Lawless, J. (1995). *The illustrated encyclopedia of essential oils.* London: Element Books Ltd.

Levine, D.P. (2006). Vancomycin: A history. *Clinical Infectious Diseases, 42,* S5-S12. doi:10.1086/491709

Levy, S. (1992). *The antibiotic paradox: How the misuse of antibiotics destroys their curative powers.* New York: Plenum Press.

Liao, F., Huang, Q., Yang, Z., Xu, H., and Gao, Q. (2004). Experimental study on the antibacterial effect of origanum volatile oil on dysentery bacilli in vivo and in vitro. *Journal of Huazhong University of Science and Technology, 24*(4), 400-403.

Mann, J. (2001). *Oil of oregano: An herbal solution to the antibiotic crisis.* Lumby, BC: Joy of the Mountains.

Manohar V., Ingram, C., Gray, J., Talpur, N.A., Echard, B.W., Bagchi, D., & Preuss, H.G. (2001). Antifungal activities of origanum oil against Candida albicans. *Molecular and Cellular Biochemistry, 228,* 111-117.

Mohacsi-Farkas, C., Tulok, M., & Balogh, B. (2003). Antimicrobial activity of Greek oregano and winter savory extracts (essential oil and SCFE) investigated by impedimetry. *Acta Horticulturae, 597,* 199-204.

Mothana, R.A., Abdo, S.A., Hasson, S., Althawab, F.M., Alaghbari, S.A., & Lindequist, U. (2010). Antimicrobial, antioxidant and cytotoxic activities and phytochemical screening of some Yemeni medicinal plants. *Evidence-Based Complementary and Alternative Medicine, 7*(3), 323-330. doi:10.1093/ecam/nen004

Natural Resources Defense Council. (2010, August 5). *Triclosan exposure levels increasing in humans, new data shows potential for food contamination* [Press release]. Retrieved from http://www.nrdc.org/

Natural Resources Defense Council. (2011). *Triclosan and triclocarban* [Chemical index]. Retrieved from http://www.nrdc.org/

Nikaido, H. (2009). Multidrug resistance in bacteria. *Annual Review of Biochemistry, 78,* 119-146. doi:10.1146/annurev.biochem.78.082907.145923

Norberg, P., Bergström, M., Jethava,V., Dubhashi, D., & Hermansson, M. (2011, April). The IncP-1 plasmid backbone adapts to different host bacterial species and evolves through homologous recombination. *Nature Communications, 2,* 68. doi:10.1038/ncomms1267

Nostro, A., Blanco, A.R., Cannatelli, M.A., Enea, V., Flamini, G., Morelli, I., . . . Alonzo, V. (2004). Susceptibility of methicillin-resistant staphylococci to oregano essential oil, carvacrol and thymol. *FEMS Microbiology Letters, 230,* 191-195.

O'Brien, T.F. (2002, June). Emergence, spread, and environmental effect of antimicrobial resistance: How use of an antimicrobial anywhere can increase resistance to any antimicrobial anywhere else. *Clinical Infectious Diseases, 34*(Supplement 3), S78-S84.

Oregano could help eradicate MRSA superbug. (2008, November 25). *The Telegraph.* Retrieved from http://www.telegraph.co.uk

Perencevich, E.N., Wong, M.T., & Harris, A.D. (2001, October). National and regional assessment of the antibacterial soap market: A step toward determining the impact of prevalent antibacterial soaps. *American Journal of Infection Control, 29*(5), 281-283.

Race against time to develop new antibiotics. (2011, February). *Bulletin of the World Health Organization, 89*, 88-89. Retrieved from http://www.who.int/

Resistance genes in our food supply. (2007, May 23). *Science Daily*. Retrieved from http://www.sciencedaily.com/

Rothberg, M.B., Haessler, S.D., & Brown, R.B. (2008, April). Complications of viral influenza. *The American Journal of Medicine, 121*(4), 258-264. doi:10.1016/j.amjmed.2007.10.040

Ruuskanen, O., Lahti, E., Jennings, L.C., & Murdoch D.R. (2011, April). Viral pneumonia. *Lancet, 377*(9773), 1264-1275. doi:10.1016/S0140-6736(10)61459-6

Rysz, M., Mansfield, W.R., Fortner, J.D., & Alvarez, P.J.J. (2013, February 5). Tetracycline resistance gene maintenance under varying bacterial growth rate, substrate and oxygen availability, and tetracycline concentration. *Environmental Science & Technology*. doi:10.1021/es3035329

Scallan, E., Griffin, P.M., Angulo, F.J., Tauxe, R.V., & Hoekstra, R.M. (2011). Foodborne illness acquired in the United States—unspecified agents. *Emerging Infectious Diseases, 17*(1), 16-22. doi:10.3201/eid1701.P21101

Schnaubelt, K. (1998). *Advanced aromatherapy*. Rochester, VT: Healing Arts Press.

Sellar, W. (2001). *The directory of essential oils*. London, England: Random House.

Shapiro, S., & Guggenheim, B. (1995). The action of thymol on oral bacteria. *Oral Microbiology and Immunology, 10*(4), 241-246.

Skandamis, P., Koutsoumanis, K., Fasseas, K., & Nychas, G-J.E. (2001). Inhibition of oregano essential oil and EDTA on Escherichia coli O157:H7. *Italian Journal of Food Science, 13*, 65-75.

Smillie, C.S., Smith, M.B., Friedman, J., Cordero, O.X., David, L.A., & Alm, E.J. (2011, December). Ecology drives a global network of gene exchange connecting the human microbiome. *Nature, 480*, 241-244. doi:10.1038/nature10571

Sokmen, M., Serkedjieva, J., Daferera, D., Gulluce, M., Polissiou, M., Tepe, B., . . . Sokmen, A. (2004). In vitro antioxidant, antimicrobial, and antiviral activities of the essential oil and various extracts from herbal parts and callus cultures of Origanum acutidens. *Journal of Agricultural and Food Chemistry, 52*(11), 3309-3312. doi:10.1021/jf049859g

Sokovic, M., Tzakou, O., Pitarokili, D., & Couladis, M. (2002). Antifungal activities of selected aromatic plants growing wild in Greece. *Die Nahrung, 46*(5), 317-320.

Soylu, S., Yigitbas, H., Soylu, E.M., & Kurt, S. (2007). Antifungal effects of essential oils from oregano and fennel on Sclerotinia sclerotiorum. *Journal of Applied Microbiology, 103*(4), 1021-1030.

Spellberg, B., Guidos, R., Gilbert, D., Bradley, J., Boucher, H.W., Scheld, W.M., . . . Infectious Diseases Society of America (IDSA). (2008). The epidemic of antibiotic-resistant infections: A call to action for the medical community from the Infectious Diseases Society of America. *Clinical Infectious Diseases, 46*(2), 155-164. doi:10.1086/524891

Subbiah, M., Shah, D.H., Besser, T.E., Ullman, J.L., & Call, D.R. (2012). Urine from treated cattle drives selection for cephalosporin resistant Escherichia coli in soil. *PLOS ONE, 7*(11), e48919. doi:10.1371/journal.pone.0048919

Tillotson, A. (2001). *The one earth herbal sourcebook.* New York: Kensington.

Ultee, A., Kets, E.P.W., & Smid, E.J. (1999). Mechanisms of action of carvacrol on the food-borne pathogen Bacillus cereus. *Applied and Environmental Microbiology, 65*(10), 4606-4610.

Ulukanli, Z., Ulukanli, S., Ozbay, H., Ilcim, A., & Tuzcu, M. (2005). Antimicrobial activities of some plants from the Eastern Anatolia Region of Turkey. *Pharmaceutical Biology, 43*, 334-339.

University of the West of England. (2008). Scientists win SEED award for Himalayan oregano

project [Press release]. Retrieved from http://info.uwe.ac.uk/

Vimalanathan, S., & Hudson, J. (2012). Anti-influenza virus activities of commercial oregano oils and their carriers. *Journal of Applied Pharmaceutical Science, 02*(07), 214-218. doi:10.7324/JAPS.2012.2734

Wilcox, J.K., Ash, S.L., & Catignani, G.L. (2004). Antioxidants and prevention of chronic disease. *Critical Reviews in Food Science and Nutrition, 44*(4), 275-295.

Wise, R. (2002). Antimicrobial resistance: Priorities for action. *Journal of Antimicrobial Chemotherapy, 49,* 585–586. doi:10.1093/jac/49.4.585

World Health Organization. (2009a). *Current WHO phase of pandemic alert for Pandemic (H1N1) 2009* [WHO Guidance Document]. Retrieved from http://www.who.int/

World Health Organization. (2009b, April 25). *Swine influenza* [Statement by WHO Director-General, Dr. Margaret Chan]. Retrieved from http://www.who.int/

World Health Organization. (2009c, April). *Influenza (seasonal)* [Fact Sheet]. Retrieved from http://www.who.int/

World Health Organization. (2011, April 6). *Antimicrobial resistance: No action today, no cure tomorrow* [Remarks by WHO Director-General, Dr. Margaret Chan]. Retrieved from http://www.who.int/

World Health Organization. (2012, March 14). *Antimicrobial resistance in the European Union and the world* [Keynote address by WHO Director-General, Dr. Margaret Chan]. Retrieved from http://www.who.int/

World Health Organization. (2013a). *Deaths from NCDs* [Global Health Observatory]. Retrieved from http://www.who.int/

World Health Organization. (2013b). *Disease outbreaks by year* [Global Alert and Response]. Retrieved from http://www.who.int/

Wright, G.D. (2012, January). Antibiotics: A new hope. *Chemistry & Biology, 19*(1), 3-10. doi:10.1016/j.chembiol.2011.10.019

Wu, T. (2011). Carbapenem-resistant or multidrug-resistant acinetobacter baumannii: A clinician's perspective. *The Hong Kong Medical Diary, Medical Bulletin, 16*(4), 6-9.

Xi, C., Zhang, Y., Marrs, C.F., Ye, W., Simon, C., Foxman, B., & Nriagu, J. (2009, September). Prevalence of antibiotic resistance in drinking water treatment and distribution systems. *Applied and Environmental Microbiology, 75*(17), 5714-5718. doi:10.1128/AEM.00382-09

Yang, J., Wang, C., Shu, C., Liu, L., Geng, J., Hu, S., & Feng, J. (2013, February 1). Marine sediment bacteria harbor antibiotic resistance genes highly similar to those found in human pathogens. *Microbial Ecology.*

Zhang, X.X., Zhang, T., & Fang, H.H. (2009, March). Antibiotic resistance genes in water environment. *Applied Microbiology and Biotechnology, 82*(3), 397-414. doi:10.1007/s00253-008-1829-z

Websites Referenced:

- Mayo Clinic
  (http://www.mayoclinic.com/)

- MEDLINE®/PubMed®
  (http://www.nlm.nih.gov/bsd/pmresources.html)

- U.S. National Library of Medicine
  (http://www.nlm.nih.gov/)

- National Institutes of Health
  (http://www.nih.gov/)

Appendix A - List of Health Conditions

Oil of Oregano may be used for the following health conditions:

Colds and Flus

- Boosts the immune system
- Combats viral and bacterial infections
- Protects you when others around you are sick
- Eases congestion in lungs and sinuses
- Relieves coughing
- Relieves sore throat

Skin Conditions

- Combats fungal, bacterial, and parasitic infections
- Heals dry and cracked skin, rashes and sores
- Reduces acne pimples and clogged pores
- Reduces swelling and pain from insect bites
- Relieves itchy skin and dandruff
- Repairs tissue and speeds healing
- May help psoriasis and eczema
- Treats foot and nail fungus
- Treats cold sores and herpes outbreaks
- Treats measles and chickenpox
- Treats ringworm, rosacea, scabies, and head lice
- Helps with shingles
- Repels mosquitos

Respiratory and Sinus Conditions

- Aids respiratory disorders and breathing difficulties
- Combats viral, bacterial, and mold infections
- Eases congestion in lungs and sinuses
- Relieves coughing
- Assists with chronic bronchitis, sinusitis, and pneumonia
- Assists with rhinitis and allergies

Sore Muscles and Joints

- Reduces pain and inflammation
- Relaxes tight muscles and spasms
- Speeds healing and improves mobility
- Alleviates arthritis, rheumatism, bursitis, tendonitis, and carpal tunnel syndrome
- Great for injuries, including sprains, strains, and torn muscles and ligaments
- Assists with muscle cramping and menstrual cramps

Burns, Wounds, Cuts, Bruises and Blisters

- Disinfects, prevents infection, and treats infection if it arises
- Reduces pain and inflammation
- Speeds healing of damaged tissue
- Reduces bruising

Mouth Conditions

- Combats bacterial infections
- Fights gum disease, recessions, and abscesses
- Relieves the pain of toothaches and fights the infection
- Disinfects mouth, cleans teeth, and freshens breath
- Treats cold sores and canker sores

Digestive Conditions

- Attacks viral, bacterial, fungal, and parasitic infections
- Combats intestinal worms and flukes
- Prevents and treats poisoning from food and water-borne pathogens
- Eases intestinal cramps and pain
- Relaxes and soothes stomach and intestinal lining
- Relieves indigestion, bloating, and gas
- Prescribed by naturopaths for IBS, colitis, and Crohn's
- Stimulates excretion of bile by liver to aid in digestion
- Combats acidity and heartburn
- Treats nausea and diarrhea

Infection-Related Conditions

Certain conditions listed below with an asterisk (*) are often infection-related, but not always. If in doubt, visit a trusted health professional for diagnosis before using Oil of Oregano for its antiviral, antibacterial, antifungal, or antiparasitic properties.

- Acne pimples and ingrown hairs
- Allergies
- Animal bites
- Arthritis*
- Athlete's foot
- Bed sores
- Bladder infections
- Boils
- Candida infections
- Canker sores
- Chronic bronchitis
- Cold sores and other herpes outbreaks
- Colds and flu
- Colitis and Crohn's*
- Dandruff*
- Diaper rash*
- Ear infections
- Fingernail and toenail fungus
- Food poisoning and water-borne illnesses
- Giardiasis
- Gum disease, recessions, and abscesses